SpringerBriefs in Ethics

Springer Briefs in Ethics envisions a series of short publications in areas such as business ethics, bioethics, science and engineering ethics, food and agricultural ethics, environmental ethics, human rights and the like. The intention is to present concise summaries of cutting-edge research and practical applications across a wide spectrum.

Springer Briefs in Ethics are seen as complementing monographs and journal articles with compact volumes of 50 to 125 pages, covering a wide range of content from professional to academic. Typical topics might include:

- Timely reports on state-of-the art analytical techniques
- A bridge between new research results, as published in journal articles, and a contextual literature review
- A snapshot of a hot or emerging topic
- In-depth case studies or clinical examples
- Presentations of core concepts that students must understand in order to make independent contributions

More information about this series at http://www.springer.com/series/10184

Elisabetta Lalumera • Stefano Fanti
Editors

Philosophy of Advanced Medical Imaging

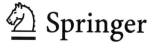 Springer

Editors
Elisabetta Lalumera
Department for Life Quality Studies
University of Bologna
Bologna, Italy

Stefano Fanti
Policlinico S. Orsola-Malpighi
University of Bologna
Bologna, Italy

ISSN 2211-8101   ISSN 2211-811X   (electronic)
SpringerBriefs in Ethics
ISBN 978-3-030-61414-0   ISBN 978-3-030-61412-6   (eBook)
https://doi.org/10.1007/978-3-030-61412-6

This Springer imprint is published by the registered company Springer Nature Switzerland AG
The registered company address is: Gewerbestrasse 11, 6330 Cham, Switzerland

Preface

This volume is a genuinely interdisciplinary work. Five of the contributors are medical doctors, specialists in nuclear medicine, five are philosophers, and two are Artificial Intelligence specialists. We, the volume editors, are a philosopher and a nuclear medicine physician. This distribution reflects our idea of what philosophy of medicine can and should be, namely, a reflection on common problems with different kinds of expertise. The risk is some heterogeneity of style in the chapters of this book, but we hope it is balanced by the interest of the contents.

We regret that for this time, we had to leave out the big topic of medical imaging and brain disorders, as we concentrated mostly on diagnostic imaging for the diagnosis of cancer.

We wish to thank all the contributors and the editorial team at Springer for their enthusiasm for this first volume on the philosophy of advanced medical imaging.

Bologna, Italy   Elisabetta Lalumera

Bologna, Italy   Stefano Fanti
August 2020

Contents

Part III Ethics

Chapter 1
The Philosophy of Advanced Medical Imaging: Mapping the Field

Elisabetta Lalumera and Stefano Fanti

Abstract The philosophy of advanced medical imaging is a new research field. Here we map the terrain with a provisional division between classical epistemology, social epistemology and ethics of advanced medical imaging. For each broad topic, we indicate what the most important questions are likely to be, review relevant samples of the existing publications, and describe the new contributions contained in this volume.

Keywords Epistemology · Ethics · Medical imaging · Diagnosis

1.1 Introduction

In the last decades, medicine has been revolutionised by advanced imaging technologies, which provided better tools for research and improved the accuracy of diagnoses. Computed tomography (CT) uses a computer to acquire a volume of X-ray based images, then reconstructed as three-dimensional pictures of inside the body, which can be rotated and viewed from any angle, providing anatomical "slices". Nuclear medicine tests such as PET use very small amounts of radioactive materials (called radiopharmaceuticals or radiotracers) to evaluate molecular, metabolic, physiologic and pathologic conditions of organs, and they can identify abnormalities very early in the progress of a disease and assess treatment response. Magnetic resonance imaging (MRI) uses a powerful magnetic field, radio frequency pulses and a computer to produce detailed pictures of organs, soft tissues, and bones. Fusion imaging may combine two imaging techniques in order to allow

E. Lalumera (✉)
Department for Life Quality Studies, University of Bologna, Bologna, Italy
e-mail: elisabetta.lalumera@unibo.it

S. Fanti
Policlinico S. Orsola-Malpighi, University of Bologna, Bologna, Italy
e-mail: stefano.fanti@aosp.bo.it

© The Author(s), under exclusive license to Springer Nature Switzerland AG 2020
E. Lalumera, S. Fanti (eds.), *Philosophy of Advanced Medical Imaging*, SpringerBriefs in Ethics, https://doi.org/10.1007/978-3-030-61412-6_1

information from two different sources to be viewed in a single set of images, such as for PET/CT. Such techniques are now widely utilised to diagnose and manage the treatment of cancer, heart disease, brain disorders such as Alzheimer's and Parkinson's disease, gastrointestinal disorders, lung disorders, bone disorders, kidney and thyroid disorders (SNMMI 2019).

What has this to do with philosophy? In fact, quite a lot. More specifically, there is a range of philosophical questions that arise in connection with advanced imaging, with diagnosis, and with the practice of radiology and nuclear medicine. The next three sections of this chapter will be aimed at mapping this terrain. Our map of the field will show three main areas – (classical) epistemology, social epistemology, and ethics – with the proviso that borders are, at least to some extent, conventional, and migration of questions from one area to the other is unavoidable. Moreover, our map will be largely one of an unexplored territory, as the interest of philosophers in advanced imaging and diagnosis is very recent, dating back one decade at most (Delehanty 2005, 2010; Lysdahl and Hofmann 2009; Hofmann 2010; Fangerau et al. 2012 with a historical perspective). In addition to the previously published literature, which is sparse, we will, therefore, refer to the chapters included in this volume, and briefly illustrate their content.

The new-born philosophy of advanced imaging can be seen as a product of diverse trends. First, recent handbooks, journal papers and edited volumes show a tendency of the philosophy of medicine of analytic tradition to move from general conceptual issues – traditionally the nature of health and disease – to special fields, such as the philosophy of evidence-based medicine, of epidemiology, pharmacology, immunology, and healthcare, to mention just a few recent examples (Solomon et al. 2016). Second, philosophers of medicine came to realise that diagnosis, in general, has been under-discussed, when compared to topics such as RCTs, placebo, or the hierarchy of evidence, and there is a research gap to be filled in this area (Stegenga et al. 2017). Finally, from the medical community, there is a request of clarification and discussion of concepts which are intrinsically value-laden and call for philosophical analysis, such as appropriateness (of a test or treatment), overtreatment, and overdiagnosis. The discussion about "Too much medicine" promoted by the British Medical Journal is an example in this sense. It brought to the forefront of the debate the need for thinking about aims and values of clinical practice when issues cannot be settled by evidence alone (BMJ 2019). In general, it is increasingly recognised that philosophers can bring a kind of expertise or skill that can be applied to questions outside traditional bioethics. Nonetheless, medical specialists call for philosophical expertise when specific ethical problems arise in everyday contexts, like the communication of a bad prognosis to an oncologic patient (Gonzalez et al. 2018).

1.2 Advanced Diagnostic Imaging and Epistemology

The main question of epistemology is: what counts as knowledge? The standard answer is the justified-true-belief account, dating back to Plato, and discussed and criticised in many ways – given a content p, a person knows that p if and only if she believes that p, she has a reason for believing that p and p is true. Epistemology of advanced diagnostic imaging turns the question to the specific domain of imaging.

Suppose a doctor reports the following, after a PET-CT scan of the patient: There are multifocal diffuse scattered hypermetabolic predominantly osteosclerotic lesions throughout the axial and proximal appendicular skeleton, compatible with widespread osseous metastases. At what conditions can we say that the doctor knows the content of the report? Her evidence is what she saw on the screen, and she formed a belief based on such evidence. When can we say that it was good, sufficient evidence? Moreover, suppose the patient reads the scan. What, if anything, counts as knowledge of the content of the report, from the patient's part? This simple example helps us introduce some broad issues in the epistemology of advanced diagnostic imaging.

1.2.1 Images as Evidence

Advanced imaging gives the illusion to see through the body. Prima facie, they provide observational evidence for a diagnostic claim. In her PhD Dissertation and a later article, Megan Delehanty (2005, 2010) investigates the peculiar nature of such observational evidence. Though they look like naturalistic images, she argues, these are rather mathematical objects, as they require several layers of mathematical and statistical processing. Her point is that the knowledge one can acquire from, say, a PET scan can qualify as knowledge from observation only if we take into account the characteristics of the technology. It is their means of production, not their similarity to body parts, what makes these images evidence. She concludes that advanced imaging – PET in particular – makes us rethink the philosophical notions of observation and empirical knowledge. Lalumera et al. (2019) elaborate on Delehanty's conclusion. They take PET as a case study and argue that it is a highly theory-laden and non-immediate knowledge procedure, despite the photographic-like quality of the images it delivers. They tackle the more general issue of what is for an advanced imaging diagnostic test to count as a reliable knowledge procedure, to which the point that follows is also related.

1.2.2   The Skill of Readers

In the sketchy example above, the doctor reports that there are lesions throughout the patient's skeleton, and these lesions are likely metastases. After investigating what is for an image counts as evidence, we need to raise the question of what makes the doctor in the position of appraising such evidence. What kind of skill or expertise does the doctor have in order to deliver the report from the image? Empirical studies in the field of medical vision tell us that expert radiologists and nuclear medicine physicians often report the sensation of knowing that a particular image contains a lesion before with a sudden "Gestalt" impression, rather than with a conscious search. On the other hand, they undergo years of intensive training that involves reading many thousands of images and learn that some areas of an organ are more likely to contain a lesion than others. Thus, eye movement recordings show that novice readers search in a relatively haphazard fashion when looking for lesions, while experienced ones tend to exhibit more concise eye movements, with fewer fixations needed to extract information (Drew et al. 2013; Friis 2017; Samei and Krupinski 2009).

Epistemology can redescribe the empirical findings with the traditional dichotomy between procedural knowledge, or knowing-how, and propositional knowledge, or knowing-that. The first is mainly unconscious and arguably direct, i.e. non-mediated by beliefs, while the latter is based on other beliefs and can be explicitly reconstructed by the knowing agent (Fantl 2017; Ryle 1971). Also, the Gestalt component of the reader's experience can be analysed by the notion of seeing-as, discussed by Ludwig Wittgenstein (2009), and a key theme in the philosophy of perception. From the epistemic point of view, these kinds of knowledge have different conditions of correctness. Once spelt out, such conditions would give a clearer picture of what counts for a doctor to know the content of a report, and the difference in performance between novice and expert readers.

1.2.3   Diagnostic Uncertainty

Even when a complete conceptual analysis of what counts as knowledge of the content of a report from the doctor's part is carried out, we still have to deal with the de facto, actual phenomenon of diagnostic uncertainty. What does it mean that the report that the doctor in our initial example communicates to the patient is uncertain? Despite the conspicuous sociological and medical literature on the topic, the concept of diagnostic uncertainty itself requires clarification (Kennedy 2017). Is uncertainty eliminable? Can there be uncertainty in the absence of error? How many kinds of uncertainty are involved in a doctor-patient encounter, in the case of advanced medical imaging?

This volume contains three original contributions by leading philosophers of medicine on diagnostic uncertainty. They are included in Part 1 of the book,

"Epistemology". In Chap. 2, "Types of diagnostic uncertainty – defining them and addressing them", Bjorn Hofmann and Kristin Bakke Lysdahl illustrate how diagnostic uncertainty can be classified according to what it is about, who experiences or scrutinises it, and which task or part of the (diagnostic) process it deals with. In conclusion, they suggest some basic rules for limiting uncertainty in practical contexts.

Ashley Graham Kennedy, in Chap. 3 ("Imaging, representation and diagnostic uncertainty") starts with arguing that medical imaging is a form of indirect observation, as we remarked above. Because of that, she argues, using an example, an image must be interpreted in the clinical context by appealing to other forms of evidence. Such an evidential pluralist strategy can mitigate the negative effects of diagnostic uncertainty.

Chapter 4, "Screening, scale and certainty", focuses on diagnostic uncertainty in screening programmes, a hotly debated topic in recent years. Stephen John uses the example of CT-based screening for lung cancer, argues that there is an epistemologically and ethically significant distinction between "individual-level" and "population-level" uncertainties, and suggests that population-level analysis should not be overlooked.

1.3 Social Epistemology of Advanced Diagnostic Imaging

Social epistemology of medicine analyses medical knowledge as a collective achievement, involving diverse subjects, institutions, scientific groups and practices. It broadens the focus of classical epistemology. A notable example of this kind of approach is Miriam Solomon's work on group decision and consensus conferences in medicine, and her book on the making of medical knowledge (Solomon 2007, 2015). This is a field where the interdisciplinary collaboration of philosophers and doctors can be particularly fruitful, as doctors have a first-person insight on the dynamics of their profession, especially if they are research leaders – for example, on the role of guidelines, of experts' meetings, on the research on radiopharmaceuticals (in nuclear medicine), on the problems of test evaluation and reliability enhancement of test, and the use of Artificial Intelligence.

Here are some examples of published literature. Lalumera et al. (2019) argued, among other points, that consensus conferences of the kind described and evaluated by Solomon are ineliminable in advanced imaging, in all those cases where the semantics of an image – the standard of interpretation – needs to be fixed. Lalumera and Fanti (2019) also illustrated the problems of evaluating the accuracy of advanced imaging diagnostic tests via randomised controlled trials, because of the nature of radiotracers, which are different from other drugs, and because RCTs inevitably end up assessing the test-plus-treatment pair, rather than the test alone. They also investigated the topic of guidelines following, by conducting qualitative research on the views of imaging experts involved in a consensus conference (Fanti et al. 2019). Finally, on the topic of shared decision making in imaging, Sophie van Baalen and

Annamaria Carusi analysed the diagnosis of Pulmonary Hypertension, including the role of advanced imaging, as a case of distributed epistemic responsibility among clinicians of various expertise and technologists, involving relations of trust (van Baalen et al. 2017; van Baalen 2019).

The section "Social Epistemology" of this volume includes three chapters, two from leading researchers in the nuclear medicine community, and one by experts of Artificial intelligence. Rodney Hicks and collaborators, in Chap. 5, "On the Inclusion of Specialists as Authors in Systematic Reviews", address the issue of the conflict, within the Evidence-based Medicine paradigm, between methodologists and clinicians in the authorship of systematic reviews. The topic is vital because systematic reviews are at the top of the hierarchy of evidence, and they provide the basis for recommendation and guidelines. Methodologists argue that clinicians are subject to self-interest as providers of healthcare services, and therefore cannot be trusted to provide unbiased guidance to either patients or policymakers. Clinicians, conversely, question whether guidelines can be formulated by individuals with neither specific expertise in medical research, nor practical experience in clinical care. They defend the reasons for clinicians with principled arguments.

John Babich and Uwe Haberkorn's Chap. 6 is on "Development of novel radiopharmaceuticals: problems, decisions and more problems". Radiopharmaceuticals or tracers are essential to the PET technique. The research on new molecules is fast-pacing and very complex. The two authors illustrate its epistemic difficulties and practical pitfalls, highlighting the choices or "Buridan's dilemmas" that the researcher is faced with, some of which are drastically underdetermined by the evidence.

The role of Artificial Intelligence and Deep Learning in advanced imaging is illustrated and assessed by Luca Casini and Marco Roccetti in Chap. 7, "Medical Imaging and Artificial Intelligence". After providing the basic notions and state of the art, Casini and Roccetti argue that Artificial intelligence and big data "open up a Pandora's box" of potential issues, including privacy and the actual responsibility of AI decision. In their conclusions, they suggest a collaboration between AI and human professionals that can leverage the best characteristics of both: "the capacity of harnessing unmanageable amounts of data to gather new insights of AI and the flexibility and specificity of the human intellect" (ibid.).

1.4 Ethical Issues in Advanced Diagnostic Imaging

Medical ethics is a vast field of study, with a long and complex tradition. Medical ethics provides normative guidance for research and clinical medicine by arguing from (ideally) universally accepted principles, such as Non-maleficence and Beneficence, Autonomy, the Utilitarian Principle, etc. In this, it is different from medical deontology, which relies on specific codes of behaviour and laws (Beauchamp and Childress 2013). Among the most discussed topics nowadays (excluding end of life and abortion) are the doctor-patient relation and the crisis of trust, the principles of Autonomy versus Paternalism, the privacy of personal data, issues related to palliative care, ethical concerns about overuse of treatments and diagnostic tests, and the ethics of communication of diagnosis (Arras 2016).

The application of ethical questions to the specific field of advanced medical imaging is to be found mostly under the label "ethics of radiology", and sample research suggests that publications tend to be in medical rather than philosophical journals (See, e.g. Barron and Kim 2003; Malone 2013). The critical questions in the ethics of radiology literature are clear once we accept that "each examination should, in theory, provide a diagnostic benefit, whether performed in the west, the developing world, the public sector or the private domain. However, each examination also represents a monetary cost and a risk, both in terms radiation exposition and other collateral damages, including the possible distress caused by an uncareful diagnosis report (IAEA 2011; Malone 2013, 108). What is the proper balance between the Principle of Beneficence and the Principle of non-Maleficence, regarding radiation exposition, and imaging testing in general? What counts as overutilisation of imaging procedures, and why is it ethically wrong? What are the ethical responsibilities of an imaging specialist in communicating a diagnosis?

This volume includes two chapters on the ethics of advanced imaging. Chapter 8 is Kristin Bakke Lysdahl and Bjorn Hofmann's "Overutilisation of imaging tests and healthcare fairness".

Overutilisation of imaging procedures is a well-known and expanding phenomenon, to be analysed not only in terms of appropriateness and cost-effectiveness but also in ethical terms. In Chap. 8, the authors define the notion, then provide a clear account of why overutilisation of diagnostic imaging is incompatible with fairness, after considering the egalitarian, the utilitarian and the contractarian notions of fairness. They also assess some potential solutions to overutilisation, including educational strategies, reinforcement of appropriateness criteria, and assigning more discretionary power to imaging specialist – which they favour as the most promising.

The last chapter of the volume is about the last passage of a medical imaging diagnostic procedure, but arguably the most crucial, namely the communication to the patient. Laetitia Marcucci and David Taieb (two professional nuclear medicine physicians) explain that there is a paucity of educational curricula on interpersonal and communication skills in imaging. Research is needed to establish ideal methods to educate professionals on communicating diagnostic imaging results, that would take into account the patients' right to decide whether they wish to receive such information or not and their right to autonomy, with personalised approaches to better integrate their capacity and vulnerability. They suggest in the conclusion that role-play scenarios could represent a solution, requiring integration of medical and philosophical expertise.

1.5   Concluding Remarks

The map of the possible exploration of the territory of intersection between advanced medical imaging and philosophy sketched so far is obviously incomplete. We are at the dawn of a new research field, and there is undoubtedly much more to come. New questions and topics of discussions will come both from philosophers to medical specialists – in order to find examples of their theorisations – but, above all, we hope, from medical specialists to philosophers, in view of human health, and of science, which requires different skills.

References

Arras, J. 2016. In *Theory and bioethics, the Stanford encyclopedia of philosophy*, ed. Edward N. Zalta, Winter 2016 ed. https://plato.stanford.edu/archives/win2016/entries/theory-bioethics/, accessed December 15, 2019.

Barron, B.J., and E.E. Kim. 2003. Ethical dilemmas in today's nuclear medicine and radiology practice. *Journal of Nuclear Medicine* 44 (11): 1818–1826.

Beauchamp, T.L., and J.F. Childress. 2013. *Principles of biomedical ethics*. USA: Oxford University Press.

British Medical Journal (BMJ) (2019). https://www.bmj.com/too-much-medicine, accessed December 28th, 2019.

Delehanty, M. 2010. Why images? *Medicine Studies* 2 (3): 161–173.

Delehanty, M.C. 2005. *Empiricism and the epistemic status of imaging technologies*. Doctoral dissertation. University of Pittsburgh.

Drew, T., K. Evans, M.L.H. Võ, F.L. Jacobson, and J.M. Wolfe. 2013. Informatics in radiology: What can you see in a single glance and how might this guide visual search in medical images? *Radiographics* 33 (1): 263–274.

Fangerau, H., R.K. Chhem, I. Müller, and S.C. Wang. 2012. *Medical imaging and philosophy*. Stuttgard: Steiner Verlag.

Fanti, S., W. Oyen, and E. Lalumera. 2019. Consensus procedures in oncological imaging: The case of prostate Cancer. *Cancers* 11 (11): 1788.

Fantl, Jeremy. 2017. In *Knowledge how. The Stanford encyclopedia of philosophy*, ed. Edward N. Zalta, Fall 2017 ed. URL =.

Friis, J. 2017. Gestalt descriptions embodiments and medical image interpretation. *AI & SOCIETY* 32 (2): 209–218.

Gonzalez, S., E. Guedj, S. Fanti, E. Lalumera, P. Le Coz, and D. Taïeb. 2018. Delivering PET imaging results to cancer patients: Steps for handling ethical issues. *European Journal of Nuclear Medicine and Molecular Imaging* 45 (12): 2240–2241.

International Atomic Energy Agency (IAEA). (2011). Radiation protection and safety of radiation sources: International basic safety standards (INTERIM EDITION). Vienna: IAEA. http://www-pub.iaea.org/MTCD/publications/PDF/p1531interim_web.pdf. Accessed 22.01.20.

Lalumera, E., and S. Fanti. 2019. Randomized controlled trials for diagnostic imaging: Conceptual and pratical problems. *Topoi* 38 (2): 395–400.

Lalumera, E., S. Fanti, and G. Boniolo. 2019. Reliability of molecular imaging diagnostics. *Synthese*: 1–17.

Lysdahl, K.B., and B.M. Hofmann. 2009. What causes increasing and unnecessary use of radiological investigations? A survey of radiologists' perceptions. *BMC Health Services Research* 9 (1): 155.

Ryle, G. 1971. [1946]. *Knowing how and knowing that.*, in Collected Papers. Vol. 2, 212–225. New York: Barnes and Nobles.

Society of Nuclear Medicine and Molecular Imaging (SNMMI) (2019), http://www.snmmi.org/AboutSNMMI/Content.aspx?ItemNumber=6433&navItemNumber=756, accessed December 28th, 2019.

Samei, E., and E. Krupinski. 2009. *The handbook of medical image perception and techniques.* Cambridge, UK: Cambridge University Press.

Solomon, M., J.R. Simon, and H. Kincaid, eds. 2016. *The Routledge companion to philosophy of medicine.* Routledge.

Stegenga, J., A. Kennedy, S. Tekin, S. Jukola, and R. Bluhm. 2017. New directions in the philosophy of medicine. In *The Bloomsbury companion to contemporary philosophy of medicine*, ed. J.A. Marcum, 343–369. London: London Bloomsbury Academic.

van Baalen, S., A. Carusi, I. Sabroe, and D.G. Kiely. 2017. A social-technological epistemology of clinical decision-making as mediated by imaging. *Journal of Evaluation in Clinical Practice* 23 (5): 949–958.

van Baalen, S.J. 2019. Knowing in medical practice: Expertise. In *Imaging technologies and interdisciplinarity.* Enschede: University of Twente. https://doi.org/10.3990/1.9789036546935.

Wittgenstein, L. 2009 [1953]. *Philosophical investigations.* London: John Wiley & Sons.

Part I
Epistemology

Chapter 2
Diagnostic Uncertainties in Medical Imaging. Analysing, Acknowledging and Handling Uncertainties in the Diagnostic Process

Bjørn Hofmann and Kristin Bakke Lysdahl

Abstract Diagnostics is a crucial tool in health care's endeavours to help people, and tremendous progress has been made in the field. Nonetheless, there are a wide range of uncertainties involved in all aspects of diagnostics – uncertainties that are important for scientific improvement, for quality of care, for practicing medicine, for informing patients, and for health policy making. In this chapter we analyse a wide range of uncertainties presenting in the various steps of diagnostic imaging. For each step we describe the main concern and suggest measures to reduce and handle the various kinds of uncertainty. Overall, we provide 9 specific measures to reduce uncertainty in the diagnostic process. Moreover, we analyse ethical issues related to the various types of uncertainty presenting at each step and end the chapter with five specific questions framed to raise the awareness of uncertainty in diagnostic imaging, as well as to reduce and to handle it. Thereby we hope that this chapter will provide practical measures to acknowledge and address diagnostic uncertainty.

Keywords Diagnostic uncertainty · Imaging · Diagnostic errors · Appropriateness

B. Hofmann (✉)
Norwegian University of Science and Technology, Gjøvik, Norway

Centre for Medical Ethics, University of Oslo, Oslo, Norway
e-mail: bjoern.hofmann@ntnu.no

K. B. Lysdahl
Faculty of Health and Social Sciences, University of South-Eastern Norway, Drammen, Norway
e-mail: Kristin.Bakke.Lysdahl@usn.no

E. Lalumera, S. Fanti (eds.), *Philosophy of Advanced Medical Imaging*, SpringerBriefs in Ethics, https://doi.org/10.1007/978-3-030-61412-6_2

2.1   Introduction

Diagnoses are crucial tools in order to help people with their existing or future suffering. However, diagnostics is not certain. There are many types of diagnostic
errors (Balogh et al. 2015), which have many sources and causes (Pinto and Brunese
2010), and a wide range of consequences (Norman and Eva 2010; Singh et al. 2017).

Defining and measuring diagnostic error is challenging (Zwaan and Singh 2015;
Hansson 2009). One crucial source of diagnostic error is diagnostic uncertainty.
Therefore, this chapter will analyse and discuss various forms of uncertainty in
diagnostics, as well as their epistemic and ethical challenges. Identifying diagnostic
uncertainties is a first step in increasing awareness of diagnostic fallibility and to
improve the quality of care and the health of individuals and populations in the long
run. Moreover, we need practical advice to how to address them. Accordingly, we
will provide five key questions and nine specific measures to address and handle the
various types of uncertainties.

2.2   Types of Uncertainty in the Diagnostic Process

There are many ways to classify and study uncertainty in the sciences in general
(Halpern 2017; Hansson 2016) and in the health sciences in particular (Hatch 2017).
In this chapter we will follow the diagnostic process in clinical practice to illustrate
the various types of diagnostic uncertainty. Table 2.1 provides an overview over the
various steps in the ordinary diagnostic process in radiology, the main concern with
each step, the corresponding issues with respect to uncertainty, and the relevant
measures to reduce uncertainty.

2.2.1   Uncertainties in Referring

In the first encounter, the health professional may be uncertain whether the patient
has a disease, what disease the patient may have, and which diagnostic test would
be appropriate. Moreover, patients and clinicians may be unaware of benefits and
risks involved in specific diagnostic examinations (Hollingsworth et al. 2019).
Clinicians may also be uncertain of the existence and relevance of referral guidelines (Greenhalgh 2013). Additionally, clinicians may be uncertainy of their own
skills in clinical examinations (Espeland and Baerheim 2003, Morgan et al. 2007),
and thus refer to radiological examinations more often than relevant. There may
also be uncertainty with respect to patient involvement in the diagnostic decision-
making process, relating patient autonomy and shared decision making
(Rogers 1919).

Table 2.1 Uncertainties, main concerns, and relevant measures to reduce uncertainty related to the various steps of the diagnostic process. Some of the uncertain issues identified at one step are also relevant for the subsequent steps

Steps	Main concern	Related uncertainty issues	Measures to reduce uncertainty
1. First encounter between patient and clinician	Appropriateness of referring	Uncertainty about the benefits and risks involved in specific diagnostic examinations	Education and training of professionals
		Uncertainty about the existence and relevance of referral guidelines	
		Clinician's uncertainty of skills in clinical examinations	
		Unclear involvement of the patient in the decision-making process (patient autonomy, shared decision making)	
2. The referral is received in the radiology department	Appropriateness of accepting test requests	Uncertainty related to unclear or missing information in the referral	Improve communication between referrer and performer.
		Unclear who is responsibility for vetting of the referral and justification of the examination	Clarify responsibility.
		Radiologists and radiographers may be uncertain about the existence or relevance of referral guidelines	Train professionals.
		Uncertain pathways for communication with referring physician	Improve communication.
3. The examination is planned and carried out	Appropriateness of test methods	Uncertainty of choice of imaging modality and procedure	Education and training of professionals.
		Unclear what responsibility the radiographer or radiologist has to supplement/correct referral information	Clarify responsibilities.
		Unclear if patients' informed consent can or should be obtained	Check with patient, medical record, or staff.
4. Review of image quality	Sufficiency of image quality	Uncertainty whether retakes are needed, due to variation in perception of image quality	Education and training of professionals.
		Uncertainty about applicable post processing	

(continued)

Table 2.1 (continued)

Steps	Main concern	Related uncertainty issues	Measures to reduce uncertainty
5. Interpretation of the images	Accuracy of diagnostic findings	Uncertainty of the accuracy of the examination (sensitivity, specificity)	Improve test quality.
		Uncertainty about the meaning of abnormalities, e.g., if very small abnormalities represent pathology (indeterminacy)	Improve interpreter skills.
		Uncertainty about pre-test probability and prevalence, and hence about the predictive value of a test result	Increase knowledge about prevalence and disease symptoms and definitions.
		Prognostic uncertainty (will it matter?)	Restrict testing with low pre-test probability.
		Uncertainty due to intra-observer and inter-observer variability.	Increase knowledge about disease progression.
6. Writhing the radiology report	Relevance of findings to report	Uncertainty of the clinical relevance of incidental finding	Increase knowledge about disease progression. Personalize medicine.
		Unclear if this relevance should be determined by the radiologist or the clinical referrer	Clarify responsibility. Align objectives of referrer and executor of the examination.
7. Providing and communicating the results to the patient	Appropriateness of communicating the findings	Lack of clarity about whether informing the patient is a task for the referring physician or the radiologist (and in some cases radiographer)	Ascetain patient autonomy, informed consent.
		Uncertainty about what "findings" to include in the information, all vs. those of clinical relevance	Ascertain shared decision-making.
		Deciding what is "clinical relevance"	Provide professional training and pay attention to professional discretion, autonomy and integrity.

Hence, in the context of the initial encounter between health professional and patient the diagnostic uncertainty is related to disease status, relevance and justification of a specific examination, and related to the diagnostic skills of the referring health professional. The main measure to reduce the uncertainties of this part of the diagnostic process is to educate and train professionals.

2.2.2 Uncertainties in Accepting Test Requests

The process of assessing the referral and deciding on what to do is subject to several types of uncertainty. First, there is uncertainty related to unclear or missing information in the referral (Davendralingam et al. 2017, Matthews and Brennan 2008). Second, it may be unclear who is responsible for vetting of the referral and for assessing justification of the examination (Vom and Williams 2017). Third, radiologists and radiographers may be uncertain about the existence or relevance of referral guidelines (Greenhalgh 2013). Fourth, there may be uncertain pathways for communication with the referring professional (Lysdahl et al. 2010). All these aspects may result in diagnostic uncertainty with respect to whether to make an examination and (in case) which examination to make.

The main measures to reduce the uncertainty related to referral assessment is to improve communication between referrer and performer, clarify responsibility, and train professionals.

2.2.3 Uncertainties in Testing Methods (Finding the Right Examination)

When it is decided that an examination is warranted, the next decision is on the right examination, e.g., the imaging modality and procedure (Djulbegovic et al. 2011). This decision may be hampered by uncertainty of the effectiveness and efficiency of a specific modality for this particular patient. The responsibility of the radiologists and radiographer with respect to supplementing/correcting referral information may also be unclear (Egan and Baird 2003), and it may be unclear if patient's informed consent can or should be obtained (Berlin 2014). To reduce these uncertainties, increase the quality of the imaging services, and the ethical standards, education and training of professionals is a crucial measure as is clarifying the responsibility of professionals.

2.2.4   Uncertainties About Image Quality

Prior to diagnosing, there may be uncertainty with respect to whether the image or examination quality is good enough for the task. There may for example be questions about whether retakes are needed due to image quality or variation in perception of image quality. Surprisingly high retake rates have been reported (Andersen et al. 2012; Waaler and Hofmann 2010; Hofmann et al. 2015), illustrating that this is a real problem. Correspondingly, there may be uncertainty about whether and what post processing is applicable (Decoster et al. 2015).

Education and training of professionals are appropriate measures to reduce such uncertainties.

2.2.5   Uncertainty About Diagnostic Findings

Once the examination is carried out, and its quality is found acceptable, a wide range of uncertainties emerge. There is uncertainty with respect to the meaning of findings, e.g., whether very small abnormalities represent pathology. This is a matter of how findings are defined, i.e., a conceptual type of uncertainty also called indeterminacy (Wynne 1992). It is uncertainty about how to define disease (Djulbegovic et al. 2011) and about using vague concepts in the description of the findings (Korsbrekke 2000).

Then there is uncertainty with respect to the accuracy of the examination (sensitivity, specificity), also called diagnostic accuracy efficacy (Fryback and Thornbury 1991). This is a question of whether the test can find abnormalities that could be found by other means (gold standard). However, even when diagnostic accuracy is known there may be uncertainty about pre-test probability and prevalence, making the predictive values of a test result uncertain. Hence, we do not know whether a positive test actually means that a patient has the disease (positive predictive value) or whether a negative test means that the person does not have the disease (negative predictive value).

However, even if the test is accurate and the test correctly identifies an underlying condition, it is not clear that this will influence the health of a person. That is, we do not know whether what we correctly find will matter in terms of causing pain and suffering. For example, if we correctly identify a precursor of disease, it is not clear that this will develop into symptoms, manifest disease, suffering, and eventually death if not detected and treated. This problem is frequently recognized as overdiagnosis (Hofmann 2014). It occurs due to uncertainty in the relationship between indicators, precursors, risk factors, disease manifestations, suffering, and death, i.e., because we do not know how these factors develop. This type of uncertainty is called prognostic uncertainty because it is temporal, and it results in overdiagnosis (Hofmann 2017, 2019a, b).

Prognostic uncertainty may have two components, development uncertainty and progression uncertainty. Progression uncertainty occurs because we do not know whether the condition which we (correctly) identify in terms of signs and symptoms

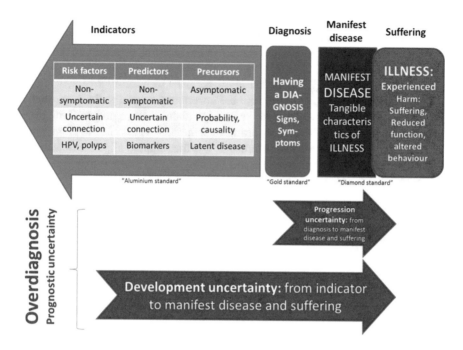

Fig. 2.1 The relationship between progression uncertainty and development uncertainty. (Adapted from Hofmann (2019a))

actually develops to manifest disease and/or death (if not detected and treated). Development uncertainty occurs because we do not know whether the risk factors, predictors, and precursors that we identify develop into signs and symptoms, manifest disease, and suffering. Figure 2.1 gives an overview of these kinds of uncertainty.

As the uncertainties with respect to diagnostic findings are diverse, so are the measures to reduce them. First and foremost, we should clarify disease definitions (Pandharipande et al. 2016), i.e., reduce indeterminacy. Then we should improve test quality and interpreter skills. Additionally, we should restrict testing with low pre-test probability and increase knowledge about disease progression. Then it is crucial to align interpreters' performance to reduce intra-observer and inter-observer variability (Korsbrekke 2000).

2.2.6   Reporting Uncertainty

When the diagnosis is made, we still face with uncertainty with respect to how much and how the findings should be reported. First, there is uncertainty of the clinical relevance of certain findings, such as incidental findings (Rosenkrantz 2017; Brown 2013) or whether the findings will make any difference in subsequent diagnostics and treatment (Djulbegovic et al. 2011). Then, it is unclear who should determine the relevance of a finding, i.e., if this relevance should be determined by the radiologist or the clinical referrer. It is a challenge for the radiologist to communicate the various types of uncertainties to the referring physician in the radiology report (Bruno et al. 2017).

In order to reduce reporting uncertainty, we need to increase knowledge about disease progression (in order to reduce the uncertainty related to findings, such as incidental findings) and to increase knowledge about disease progression, i.e., to personalize medicine. To reduce reporting vagueness, it is important to align reporting language (Korsbrekke 2000). Moreover, it is important to align the objective of the examination of the referrer and the radiologist (e.g., where they are on the Receiver Operator Characteristic (ROC) curve.

2.2.7 Communication Uncertainty

There are several types of uncertainties related to providing and communicating results to the patient. First, it can be unclear if informing the patient is a task for the referring physician or the radiologist (and in some cases radiographer). Second, there may be uncertainty about what "findings" to include in the information, all vs. those of clinical relevance, for example how much to inform patients about incidental findings (Phillips et al. 2015; Kang et al. 2016). Third, there is uncertainty in deciding what is "clinical relevance," i.e., what is important. This is a type of indeterminacy, as discussed above.

As before, the ethical principles of beneficence and non-maleficence are relevant to avoid harm and ascertain the best interest of the patient. Moreover, communication uncertainty involves patient autonomy and informed consent. However, it also encompasses professional autonomy and integrity.

To reduce communication uncertainty, we may clarify responsibilities, as well as core concepts such as "clinical relevance." Additionally, shared decision-making (SDM) may be a valuable tool (Berlin 2014; Birkeland 2016; Lumbreras et al. 2017). Moreover, strengthening professional integrity and communication skills is of utmost importance. However, it is important that referrers (GPs and others) and performers (radiologists and others) may have different goals. A referring physician may want to rule out a certain condition while a radiologist may be eager not to miss any pathology (Korsbrekke 2000). Hence, the uncertainty stemming from different goals may be mitigated by clear communication between referrer and performer.

2.3 Relevance and Implications

Above we have presented various types of uncertainty related to the diagnostic process. We have also highlighted the issues related to each step, and various measures to reduce uncertainty. There are of course many other ways to classify and discuss diagnostic uncertainty in radiology. Our framework is by no means the only or the best way to do so, but it is chosen because of its familiarity to clinicians. Moreover, it can easily be related to other frameworks, which we will show in the following Thereafter we will present different perspective and conceptions of uncertainty in which diagnostic uncertainty is situated. Finally, we will address ethical issues and principles relevant for addressing diagnostic imaging uncertainties.

2.3.1   Frameworks for Uncertainty

One framework for analysing uncertainty differentiates between risk, fundamental uncertainty, ignorance, and indeterminacy (Van Asselt 2000; Wynne 1992). Risk is when you know certain outcomes and the chance that they occur. Given certain findings on the image, you know the risk that the patient has a given diagnosis. With fundamental uncertainty (also known as severe or Knightian uncertainty) you still know about the outcome (e.g., a given diagnosis) but you do not know the probability (distribution). Ignorance are unknown factors that are relevant for the diagnostic process, but which the health professional is not aware of. Indeterminacy, which formally is a type of model validity uncertainty, is uncertainty stemming from different ways to classify the conditions to be diagnosed.

Table 2.2 gives an overview of these four types of uncertainty applied to the diagnostic process discussed above.

Table 2.2 Four types of uncertainty classified according to outcomes and risks. Adapted from Stirling (2010)

Possibilities Probability	Known outcome	Unknown outcome
Known probability	**Risk**	**Indeterminacy** (ambiguity)
	Test accuracy (sensitivity, specificity, predictive values) for the various examinations in different contexts.	How to define specific findings
	Outcomes and harms of various examinations	Defining disease entities
	Knowledge about diseases (including prognosis where probabilities are known)	Vagueness in description of findings or in reporting
		Defining clinical relevance
Unknown probability	**Fundamental** (Knightian) **uncertainty**	**Ignorance**
	Prognostic uncertainty	Unknown meaning of certain markers for diagnosis or prognosis
	Development uncertainty	Unknown effects of ionizing radiation (good or bad)
	Progression uncertainty	Unknown relevance of individual health data
	Overdiagnosis, underdiagnosis	
	Value of incidental findings	

Our classification of uncertainties also corresponds with Sven Ove Hansson's early framework (Hansson 1996), which distinguishes between four general types of uncertainty, i.e., uncertainty about (i) alternatives, (ii) consequences, (iii) trustworthiness of information, and (iv) about values and conceptions amongst decision makers. Uncertainty with respect to which alternatives and consequences with respect to which diagnostic method to apply is covered by our step 3 and 4. The issue of whether the information is trustworthy is covered in step 5. Uncertainty about values and conceptions amongst decision makers, Hanson's fourth type, is covered in our 2, 6, and 7.

Correspondingly, our description of diagnostic uncertainties also correspond to other conceptions of uncertainty in a clinical setting, such as discussed by Trisha Greenhalgh (Greenhalgh 2013). Greenhalgh specifically refers to uncertainty about the specific illness narrative, about case-based reasoning (our step 2), about what the guidelines show (step 1 and 2), what best to do in the circumstances (step 3–5), about multi-professional working (step 2 and 6), and how best to communicate and collaborate (step 2, 6, and 7).

2.3.2   Different Perspectives on Uncertainty

Our approach also is informed by the ways that uncertainty is conceptualized and investigated in various academic disciplines (Han et al. 2019). In behavioural economics many see uncertainty as an obstacle to rational decision making. In clinical medicine and health services research it may be an issue of optimal evidence-based care. Psychologists may think of uncertainty as a barrier or facilitator to the satisfaction of fundamental human needs, and cognitive scientists see it as a perceptual state, and in communication science uncertainty is a product of information exchange. Moreover, in anthropology and sociology it may be viewed as a socially constructed, negotiated, and shared understanding or set of meanings (Han et al. 2019).

Uncertainty is also scrutinized in terms of vagueness, and classified in terms of linguistic vagueness, epistemic vagueness, semantic vagueness, and ontic vagueness (Sadegh-Zadeh 2012).

Paul Han defines «uncertainty as the subjective consciousness of ignorance. As such, uncertainty is a "metacognition"—a thinking about thinking—characterized by self-awareness of incomplete knowledge about some aspect of the world." (Han 2013). Han provides an overview of different conceptions of uncertainty in medicine (Han et al. 2011), which is useful for setting diagnostic uncertainty in context. See Fig. 2.2.

Han's conceptions of uncertainty relate to other classifications of uncertainty, such as indeterminacy, ignorance, unreliability, parameter uncertainty, and inexactness (Strand and Oughton 2009).

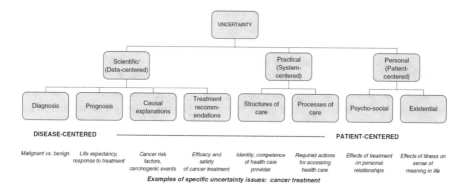

Fig. 2.2 Different conceptions and sources of uncertainty from Han et al. (2011)

2.4 Ethical Issues in Diagnostic Uncertainties

The various types of uncertainty raise a series of ethical issues, which will briefly be discussed in the following.

Two ethical principles that are relevant for all steps of the process and their related types of uncertainty are beneficence and non-maleficence (Beauchamp and Childress 2019). This should not come as a surprize as the overall aim of diagnostic imaging is to promote good for the patients and avoid harming them, and uncertainties in the diagnostic process may hamper or undermine gaining this goal. In the initial steps (1 and 2) uncertainty is mainly about whether or not the radiological examination is warranted i.e. justifiable. In step 3 and 4 decisions may be hampered by uncertainty of the effectiveness and efficiency of a specific modality or procedure or the sufficiency of the image quality for the particular patient (e.g. based on insufficient referral information). All such uncertainties can obviously lead to wrong decisions and cause suboptimal examinations, which in turn may compromise patients' benefit in terms of reduced probability of a correct diagnosis and subsequent treatment as well as exposing patients to unnecessary risks of harm, i.e., reduced safety. Uncertainties that occur later in the process may also fail to promote benefits to the patient and/or cause harm due to inaccuracy or irrelevant findings. False-negative finding are for instance the major contributor to patient injury compensation claims in radiology (Bose et al. 2019). Likewise, is it of crucial importance not to harm the patient by causing unnecessary subsequent examination or treatments, or anxiety due to irrelevant information. This means that the principles of beneficence and non-maleficence urge us to avoid inaccurate, false or incidental findings, and overdiagnosis (Mendelson and Montgomery 2016), followed by inappropriate patient management and follow-up procedures that are invasive, risky and expensive (Burger and Kass 2009).

The principles of justice and solidarity are relevant as uncertainties here may lead to misuse, underuse and overuse of services. For example, uncertainties about appropriateness of referring the patient and accepting the referral (step 1 and 2), challenge justice and solidarity (see Chap. 8: Overutilization of imaging tests and healthcare fairness). Justice is also relevant more indirectly in the rest of the process due to the incorrect decisions and the subsequent waste of resources based on uncertainties.

The principle respect for patients' autonomy and as well as dignity is relevant in step 1 regarding the uncertainties in involving the patient in decision-making process. This is a challenging task for the clinician as patients demand for imaging services is an important driver for inappropriate imaging (Hendee et al. 2010). The uncertainty may easily occur in cases when the patient wants an examination for other the strictly medical reasons and respecting the patient's autonomy and dignity becomes incompatible with following best practice. In step 3 the relevance of patient autonomy regards the radiographers' uncertainty about if and how informed consent can or should be obtained (Younger et al. 2019). Moreover, patient autonomy is also involved in step 5 and 6 because it is crucial to inform patients about the types of uncertainty that should be considered along the results (Hofmann and Lysdahl 2008).

Professional autonomy, accountability, responsibility, and/or integrity are relevant aspects in many steps in the diagnostic process for the obvious reason that professionals are the main actors in the process. For instance, in step 1 the uncertainties in skills in clinical examination (Espeland and Baerheim 2003; Morgan et al. 2007) and ignorance about clinical referral guidelines (Gransjoen et al. 2018), clearly raise questions about professionals' integrity and responsibility. Adherence to guidelines may be perceived incompatible with professional autonomy. Similar arguments can be made for step 2: the uncertainties related to justification or examinations (Vom and Williams 2017) and communication challenges (Strudwick and Day 2014) call for the professionals' responsibility.

Correspondingly, uncertainty raise issues of professional integrity and autonomy in decision making in step 3 and 4 as well as issues of the distribution of responsibility between professionals, e.g. regarding improvement of the referral information (Lam et al. 2004) and determining sufficient image quality (Mount 2016).

In the final step of the diagnostic process, the radiologists bear a heavy load of responsibility for dealing with the uncertainty inherent in the process of interpreting and reporting the radiological findings (Bruno 2017), for instance the challenges related to incidentalomas (Berlin 2013), and uncertainties in patient information responsibilities (Gutzeit et al. 2019). For more general treatments of ethics and responsibility of science and technology, see (Hansson 2003, 2013; Fahlquist 2018).

2.5 Handling Diagnostic Uncertainty

We have provided an overview of the various ethical aspects and measures to reduce uncertainty at 7 steps of diagnosis. Summarising these (given in the right column of Table 2.1) gives us 9 specific measures to reduce uncertainty in the diagnostic process:

Educate and train professionals, especially in performance and interpreting skills
Improve communication between referrer and performer and to the patient.
Clarify the responsibility for the various acts and agents in all the steps of the diagnostic process.

Clarify definitions of findings, diagnoses, and diseases

Be cautious when the prevalence is low and restrictive when the pre-test probability is low

Increase knowledge about disease progression and individual variability

Increase knowledge about disease prognostics

Communicate uncertainty to patients and apply shared decision-making

Strengthen professional integrity

One important topic expected to influence diagnostic uncertainties in diagnostic imaging and the way they can be handled is artificial intelligence (AI). This is a too big an issue to address fully in this chapter. Suffice here is to point out that AI may reduce the uncertainties discussed in steps 2–5, and subsequently also in 6 and 7. However, introducing AI in order to improve diagnostics and reduce uncertainty also introduces two important and related challenges: the black box problem and responsibility.

AI introduces algorithms that are non-explanatory ("the black box problem"), which makes it difficult to understand why a certain diagnosis or decision is reached. This then makes it difficult to distribute responsibility (Neri et al. 2020; Pesapane et al. 2018). Who is responsible for a decision based on an AI-provided diagnosis that turns out to be wrong? Is it the AI-constructor or vender? The provider of the data on which the AI-system is trained or used? The health care system implementing the AI-system? The professional using it? Or the patient consenting to its use? These issues merit a separate paper.

If we focus on the overall goal of diagnostics, i.e., to find the underlying and potentially modifiable cause of pain and suffering (in terms of disease) and thereby to help people, we can boil the advice to handle diagnostic uncertainty down to five key questions:

1. Is it right to test? (Appropriateness of testing)
2. Is it the right test? (Test appropriateness)
3. Is the test right? (Accuracy of result, trustworthiness)
4. Is the test clinically helpful? (Relevance of result)
5. Does the test result matter to the patient? (Importance of result)

Figure 2.3 presents the five steps to handle diagnostic uncertainty in practice.

Addressing these questions will make it easier to handle uncertainty and improve diagnostics in radiology.

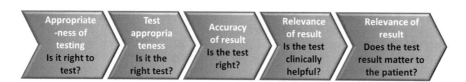

Fig. 2.3 Five basic issues and questions to ask in order to reduce diagnostic uncertainty. (Adapted from Hofmann (2018))

2.6   Conclusion

In this chapter we have analysed a wide range of uncertainties presenting in seven steps of diagnostic imaging. For each step we have described the main concern and suggested measures to reduce and handle the various kinds of uncertainty. Overall, we have provided 9 specific measures to reduce uncertainty in the diagnostic process. Moreover, we have analysed ethical issues related to the various types of uncertainty presenting at each step of the diagnostic process and discussed the ethical principles relevant for addressing these issues. We have also demonstrated how the uncertainties presented and discussed in this chapter relate to the general literature on uncertainty and briefly indicated how AI may change and challenge diagnostic uncertainty. We ended this chapter with five specific questions framed to raise the awareness of uncertainty in diagnostic imaging, as well as to reduce and to handle it. Thereby we hope that this chapter provide practical measures to acknowledge and address diagnostic uncertainty.

References

Andersen, E.R., J. Jorde, N. Taoussi, S.H. Yaqoob, B. Konst, and T. Seierstad. 2012. Reject analysis in direct digital radiography. *Acta Radiologica* 53 (2): 174–178. https://doi.org/10.1258/ar.2011.110350.

Balogh, Erin P., Bryan T. Miller, John R. Ball, and Engineering National Academies of Sciences, and Medicine. 2015. Overview of diagnostic error in health care. In *Improving diagnosis in health care*. Washington, DC: National Academies Press.

Beauchamp, T.L., and J.F. Childress. 2019. *Principles of biomedical ethics*. New York: Oxford University Press New York.

Berlin, L. 2013. MEDICOLEGAL: Malpractice and ethical issues in radiology: The incidentaloma. *AJR. American Journal of Roentgenology* 200 (1): W91. https://doi.org/10.2214/AJR.12.8894.

Berlin, Leonard. 2014. Shared decision-making: Is it time to obtain informed consent before radiologic examinations utilizing ionizing radiation? Legal and ethical implications. *Journal of the American College of Radiology* 11 (3): 246–251.

Birkeland, Søren. 2016. Shared decision making in interventional radiology. *Radiology* 278 (1): 302–303.

Bose, A.M., I.R. Khan Bukholm, G. Bukholm, and J.T. Geitung. 2019. A national study of the causes, consequences and amelioration of adverse events in the use of MRI, CT, and conventional radiography in Norway. *Acta Radiologica* 61: 284185119881734. https://doi.org/10.1177/0284185119881734.

Brown, Stephen D. 2013. Professional norms regarding how radiologists handle incidental findings. *Journal of the American College of Radiology* 10 (4): 253–257.

Bruno, M.A. 2017. 256 shades of gray: Uncertainty and diagnostic error in radiology. *Diagnosis* 4 (3): 149–157. https://doi.org/10.1515/dx-2017-0006.

Bruno, M.A., J. Petscavage-Thomas, and H.H. Abujudeh. 2017. Communicating uncertainty in the radiology report. *AJR. American Journal of Roentgenology* 209 (5): 1006–1008. https://doi.org/10.2214/AJR.17.18271.

Burger, I.M., and N.E. Kass. 2009. Screening in the dark: Ethical considerations of providing screening tests to individuals when evidence is insufficient to support screening populations. *The American Journal of Bioethics* 9 (4): 3–14.

Davendralingam, N., M. Kanagaratnam, L. Scarlett, M. Moor, P. MacCallum, and E. Friedman. 2017. An audit on the appropriateness of information provided on DVT US requests for suitable vetting and justification. *Clinical Radiology* 72 (Supplement 1): S20.

Decoster, R., H. Mol, and D. Smits. 2015. Post-processing, is it a burden or a blessing? Part 1 evaluation of clinical image quality. *Radiography* 21 (1): e1–e4.

Djulbegovic, Benjamin, Iztok Hozo, and Sander Greenland. 2011. Uncertainty in clinical medicine. *Philosophy of Medicine* 16: 299.

Egan, I., and M. Baird. 2003. Optimising the diagnostic imaging process through clinical history documentation. *The Radiographer* 50 (1): 11–18.

Espeland, A., and A. Baerheim. 2003. Factors affecting general practitioners' decisions about plain radiography for back pain: Implications for classification of guideline barriers–A qualitative study. *BMC Health Services Research* 3 (1): 8.

Fahlquist, Jessica Nihlén. 2018. *Moral responsibility and risk in society: Examples from emerging technologies*. Routledge: Public Health and Environment.

Fryback, Dennis G., and John R. Thornbury. 1991. The efficacy of diagnostic imaging. *Medical Decision Making* 11 (2): 88–94.

Gransjoen, A.M., S. Wiig, K.B. Lysdahl, and B.M. Hofmann. 2018. Barriers and facilitators for guideline adherence in diagnostic imaging: An explorative study of GPs' and radiologists' perspectives. *BMC Health Services Research* 18 (1): 556. https://doi.org/10.1186/s12913-018-3372-7.

Greenhalgh, Trisha. 2013. Uncertainty and clinical method. In *Clinical uncertainty in primary care*, 23–45. New York: Springer.

Gutzeit, A., R. Heiland, S. Sudarski, J.M. Froehlich, K. Hergan, M. Meissnitzer, S. Kos, P. Bertke, O. Kolokythas, and D.M. Koh. 2019. Direct communication between radiologists and patients following imaging examinations. Should radiologists rethink their patient care? *European Radiology* 29 (1): 224–231. https://doi.org/10.1007/s00330-018-5503-2.

Halpern, Joseph Y. 2017. *Reasoning about uncertainty*. Cambridge, MA: MIT press.

Han, Paul K.J. 2013. Conceptual, methodological, and ethical problems in communicating uncertainty in clinical evidence. *Medical Care Research and Review* 70 (1 suppl): 14S–36S.

Han, Paul K.J., William M.P. Klein, and Neeraj K. Arora. 2011. Varieties of uncertainty in health care: A conceptual taxonomy. *Medical Decision Making* 31 (6): 828–838.

Han, P.K.J., A. Babrow, M.A. Hillen, P. Gulbrandsen, E.M. Smets, and E.H. Ofstad. 2019. Uncertainty in health care: Towards a more systematic program of research. *Patient Education and Counseling* 102 (10): 1756–1766. https://doi.org/10.1016/j.pec.2019.06.012.

Hansson, Sven Ove. 1996. Decision making under great uncertainty. *Philosophy of the Social Sciences* 26 (3): 369–386.

———. 2003. Ethical criteria of risk acceptance. *Erkenntnis* 59 (3): 291–309.

———. 2009. Measuring uncertainty. *Studia Logica* 93 (1): 21–40.

———. 2013. *The ethics of risk: Ethical analysis in an uncertain world*. Dordrecht: Springer.

———. 2016. Evaluating the uncertainties. In *The argumentative turn in policy analysis*, 79–104. London: Springer.

Hatch, Steven. 2017. Uncertainty in medicine. *BMJ* 357: 1713. https://doi.org/10.1136/bmj.j2180. https://www.bmj.com/content/bmj/357/bmj.j2180.full.pdf.

Hendee, W.R., G.J. Becker, J.P. Borgstede, J. Bosma, W.J. Casarella, B.A. Erickson, C.D. Maynard, J.H. Thrall, and P.E. Wallner. 2010. Addressing overutilization in medical imaging. *Radiology* 257 (1): 240–245. https://doi.org/10.1148/radiol.10100063.

Hofmann, Bjørn. 2014. Diagnosing overdiagnosis: Conceptual challenges and suggested solutions. *European Journal of Epidemiology* 29 (9): 599–604. https://doi.org/10.1007/s10654-014-9920-5. http://www.kunnskapssenteret.no/publikasjoner/langtidseffekter-etter-fedmekirurgi.

Hofmann, B. 2017. Overdiagnostic uncertainty. *European Journal of Epidemiology* 32 (6): 533–534. https://doi.org/10.1007/s10654-017-0260-0.

―――. 2018. Looking for trouble? Diagnostics expanding disease and producing patients. *Journal of Evaluation in Clinical Practice* 24 (5): 978–982. https://doi.org/10.1111/jep.12941.

―――. 2019a. Back to basics: Overdiagnosis is about unwarranted diagnosis. *American Journal of Epidemiology* 188: 1812–1817. https://doi.org/10.1093/aje/kwz148.

―――. 2019b. Overdiagnosis: Epistemic uncertainty and ethical challenges. *BMJ Evidence-Based Medicine* 24: A11.

Hofmann, Bjørn, and Kristin Bakke Lysdahl. 2008. Moral principles and medical practice: The role of patient autonomy in the extensive use of radiological services. *Journal of Medical Ethics* 39: 446–449. https://doi.org/10.1136/jme.2006.019307. http://jme.bmjjournals.com/.

Hofmann, Bjørn, Tina Blomberg Rosanowsky, Camilla Jensen, and Kenneth Wah. 2015. Image rejects in general direct digital radiography. *Acta Radiologica Open* 4 (10): 1–6.

Hollingsworth, T.D., R. Duszak Jr., A. Vijayasarathi, R.B. Gelbard, and M.E. Mullins. 2019. Trainee knowledge of imaging appropriateness and safety: Results of a series of surveys from a large academic Medical Center. *Current Problems in Diagnostic Radiology* 48 (1): 17–21. https://doi.org/10.1067/j.cpradiol.2017.10.007.

Kang, Stella K., Kayte Spector-Bagdady, Arthur L. Caplan, and R. Scott Braithwaite. 2016. Exome and genome sequencing and parallels in radiology: Searching for patient-centered management of incidental and secondary findings. *Journal of the American College of Radiology* 13 (12): 1467–1472.

Korsbrekke, K. 2000. On radiology and radiologic method--cooperation between clinician and radiologist. *Tidsskrift for den Norske Lægeforening* 120 (16): 1907.

Lam, D., I. Egan, and M. Baird. 2004. The Radiographer's impact on improving clinical decision-making, patient care and patient diagnosis: A pilot study. *Radiographer* 51 (3): 133–137. https://doi.org/10.1002/j.2051-3909.2004.tb00012.x.

Lumbreras, Blanca, José Vilar, Isabel González-Álvarez, Mercedes Guilabert, María Pastor-Valero, Lucy Anne Parker, Jorge Vilar-Palop, and Ildefonso Hernández-Aguado. 2017. Avoiding fears and promoting shared decision-making: How should physicians inform patients about radiation exposure from imaging tests? *PLoS One* 12 (7): e0180592.

Lysdahl, K.B., B.M. Hofmann, and A. Espeland. 2010. Radiologists' responses to inadequate referrals. *European Radiology* 20 (5): 1227–1233. https://doi.org/10.1007/s00330-009-1640-y.

Matthews, K., and P.C. Brennan. 2008. Justification of x-ray examinations: General principles and an Irish perspective. *Radiography* 14 (4): 349–355.

Mendelson, R.M., and B.D. Montgomery. 2016. Towards appropriate imaging: Tips for practice. *Australian Family Physician* 45 (6): 391–395.

Morgan, M., L. Jenkins, and L. Ridsdale. 2007. Patient pressure for referral for headache: A qualitative study of GPs' referral behaviour. *British Journal of General Practice* 57 (534): 29–35.

Mount, J. 2016. Reject analysis: A comparison of radiographer and radiologist perceptions of image quality. *Radiography* 22 (2): e112–e117. https://doi.org/10.1016/j.radi.2015.12.001.

Neri, Emanuele, Francesca Coppola, Vittorio Miele, Corrado Bibbolino, and Roberto Grassi. 2020. *Artificial intelligence: Who is responsible for the diagnosis?* New York: Springer.

Norman, Geoffrey R., and Kevin W. Eva. 2010. Diagnostic error and clinical reasoning. *Medical Education* 44 (1): 94–100.

Pandharipande, Pari V., Brian R. Herts, Richard M. Gore, William W. Mayo-Smith, H. Benjamin Harvey, Alec J. Megibow, and Lincoln L. Berland. 2016. Rethinking normal: Benefits and risks of not reporting harmless incidental findings. *Journal of the American College of Radiology* 13 (7): 764–767.

Pesapane, Filippo, Caterina Volonté, Marina Codari, and Francesco Sardanelli. 2018. Artificial intelligence as a medical device in radiology: Ethical and regulatory issues in Europe and the United States. *Insights Into Imaging* 9 (5): 745–753.

Phillips, John P., Caitlin Cole, John P. Gluck, Jody M. Shoemaker, Linda E. Petree, Deborah L. Helitzer, Ronald M. Schrader, and Mark T. Holdsworth. 2015. Stakeholder opinions and ethical perspectives support complete disclosure of incidental findings in MRI research. *Ethics & Behavior* 25 (4): 332–350.

Pinto, Antonio, and Luca Brunese. 2010. Spectrum of diagnostic errors in radiology. *World Journal of Radiology* 2 (10): 377.

Rogers, W.A. 1919. Whose autonomy? Which choice? A study of GPs' attitudes towards patient autonomy in the management of low back pain. *Family Practice* 2: 140–145.

Rosenkrantz, Andrew B. 2017. Differences in perceptions among radiologists, referring physicians, and patients regarding language for incidental findings reporting. *American Journal of Roentgenology* 208 (1): 140–143.

Sadegh-Zadeh, Kazem. 2012. *Handbook of analytic philosophy of medicine*. Dordrecht: Springer.

Singh, Hardeep, Gordon D. Schiff, Mark L. Graber, Igho Onakpoya, and Matthew J. Thompson. 2017. The global burden of diagnostic errors in primary care. *BMJ Quality and Safety* 26 (6): 484–494.

Stirling, Andy. 2010. Keep it complex. *Nature* 468 (7327): 1029.

Strand, Roger, and Deborah Oughton. 2009. Risk and uncertainty as a research ethics challenge. *National Committees for Research Ethics in Norway* 9: 1–41.

Strudwick, R.M., and J. Day. 2014. Interprofessional working in diagnostic radiography. *Radiography* 20 (3): 235–240. https://doi.org/10.1016/j.radi.2014.03.009.

Van Asselt, Marjolein B.A. 2000. *Perspectives on uncertainty and risk*, 407–417. New York: Springer.

Vom, J., and I. Williams. 2017. Justification of radiographic examinations: What are the key issues? *Journal of Medical Radiation Sciences* 11: 11. https://doi.org/10.1002/jmrs.211.

Waaler, D., and B. Hofmann. 2010. Image rejects/retakes--radiographic challenges. *Radiation Protection Dosimetry* 139 (1–3): 375–379. https://doi.org/10.1093/rpd/ncq032.

Wynne, Brian. 1992. Uncertainty and environmental learning: Reconceiving science and policy in the preventive paradigm. *Global Environmental Change* 2 (2): 111–127.

Younger, C.W.E., S. Moran, C. Douglas, and H. Warren-Forward. 2019. Barriers and pathways to informed consent for ionising radiation imaging examinations: A qualitative study. *Radiography* 25 (4): e88–e94.

Zwaan, Laura, and Hardeep Singh. 2015. The challenges in defining and measuring diagnostic error. *Diagnosis* 2 (2): 97–103.

Chapter 3
Imaging, Representation and Diagnostic Uncertainty

Ashley Graham Kennedy

Abstract In recent years there has been a rapid increase in the number of diagnostic imaging tests performed by clinicians. However, the results of medical imaging tests – even highly accurate ones- are alone not enough to make accurate diagnoses in the clinical setting. Instead, careful interpretation of these results is required. When diagnostic interpretation is not done properly, this can lead to either overdiagnosis or underdiagnosis, both of which are epistemic problems that have negative practical and ethical implications for patients and clinicians, whereas proper interpretation can mitigate these diagnostic errors. Thus, it is important to understand how to handle diagnostic uncertainty regarding medical imaging. In particular, I argue that this requires both that we understand medical images as indirect representations and that we be evidential pluralists in the clinical setting. This means that what counts as evidence towards a diagnosis is not just an accurate diagnostic test or image, but a carefully interpreted diagnostic result that takes into account all of the available clinical evidence.

Keywords Diagnostic uncertainty · Overdiagnosis · Underdiagnosis · Interpretation · Evidential pluralism

3.1 Introduction

Although the use of diagnostic imaging in the clinical setting has increased rapidly in recent years, uncertainty regarding how to interpret these medical imaging tests is common. In what follows I will argue that this uncertainty, if not carefully

A. G. Kennedy (✉)
Honors College, Florida Atlantic University, Jupiter, FL, USA
e-mail: kennedya@fau.edu

approached, can in turn lead to increased rates of both overdiagnosis and underdiagnosis. Overdiagnosis and underdiagnosis are, as we will see, epistemic problems with negative pragmatic and ethical implications. Because of this, we want to avoid both situations in medical practice and therefore it is important to understand how to approach diagnostic uncertainty regarding medical imaging and how to manage it carefully in the clinical setting.

To begin, it is helpful to acknowledge that diagnostic uncertainty generally, and in regards to diagnostic medical imaging particularly, is, at present, an unavoidable part of clinical medicine. And while there are ongoing efforts to reduce this epistemic uncertainty by improving our diagnostic test accuracy, it is unlikely that this uncertainty will be completely eliminated, at least not anytime soon. I will argue, in the example that follows, that the medical image alone is never enough for an accurate diagnosis, no matter how accurate a representation it is. Instead, this image, because it is a form of indirect observation, must be interpreted in the clinical context by appeal to other forms of evidence. In other words, although the epistemic situation of diagnostic uncertainty in many instances cannot be avoided completely, it is still possible to approach it strategically in order to avoid (or at least mitigate) negative outcomes for both patients and clinicians. Some of these potential negative outcomes that can arise from mismanaged diagnostic uncertainty in the clinical setting include the epistemic (in the form of overdiagnosis or underdiagnosis), the pragmatic (in the form of increased financial and time costs), and the ethical (in the form of increased patient suffering). More specifically, both overdiagnosis and underdiagnosis can increase clinical costs as well as patient suffering, and thus we should aim to avoid them whenever possible. One way to do this is to properly interpret diagnostic imaging tests in the clinical context.

3.2 Overdiagnosis

Overdiagnosis is currently much discussed in the medical literature: the BMJ even recently devoted an entire issue to the topic. However, precisely what the term means is not currently agreed upon. Some (Rogers and Mintzker 2016) have argued that the term "refers to diagnosis that does not benefit patients because the diagnosed condition is not a harmful disease in those individuals." Others consider an "overdiagnosis" to be a diagnosis that "will not lead to an overall benefit to the patient," or that makes "people patients unnecessarily" (Broderson et al. 2018), while still others argue that, "in overdiagnosis we diagnose something that is not disease," or in other words that, "cases of overdiagnosis are not cases of disease. They are unwarranted labelling of disease" Hofmann (2017).

Following along these lines, I will use the term "overdiagnosis" to refer to the diagnosis of a patient with a condition that is not currently causing the patient to suffer and will not cause the patient to suffer if left undiagnosed.

3.3 Underdiagnosis

On the opposite end of the spectrum from overdiagnosis, is underdiagnosis, which can be understood as the phenomenon of either not diagnosing a condition at all ("missed" diagnosis) or incorrectly diagnosing ("misdiagnosis") a condition in a patient. Underdiagnosis thus often results in increased (in terms of time spent and/ or intensity of) suffering in the patient, and therefore it too, like overdiagnosis, has both negative pragmatic and ethical implications. While it is easy to see how over-diagnosis, especially when it leads to excessive testing or overtreatment, can be financially costly as well as time consuming, this is also true of underdiagnosis. For example, significant amounts of time and money (on repeated hospital or clinic visits and/or unnecessary tests and medications) are often wasted in cases of under-diagnosis. The goal then should of course be to avoid both over- and under-diagnosis and their negative implications. While this is easier said than done, there are avail-able clinical methods that can be used to facilitate this. The one that I will discuss in what follows is the recognition, as well as the appropriate handling of, the diagnos-tic uncertainty that often arises surrounding the question of how to interpret medical imaging tests. In order to facilitate this discussion I will begin with the examination of a case study.

3.4 Case Study: Arachnoid Cysts

Arachnoid cysts are fluid-filled sacs that can occur either on the arachnoid mem-brane that covers the brain (intracranial arachnoid cyst) or on the spinal cord. The most common locations for intracranial arachnoid cysts are the middle fossa (near the temporal lobe), the suprasellar region (near the third ventricle) and the posterior fossa, which contains the cerebellum, pons, and medulla oblongata. In many cases, arachnoid cysts do not cause symptoms. However, in cases in which symptoms do occur, headaches, seizures and abnormal accumulation of excessive cerebrospinal fluid in the brain (hydrocephalus) are common.

A diagnosis of arachnoid cysts is often made incidentally, most commonly dur-ing a diagnostic workup for seizures. In other cases, the diagnosis of an arachnoid cyst may be suspected based upon a patient history and a clinical examination, and subsequently confirmed by either computed tomography (CT scan) or magnetic resonance imaging (MRI). CT scans and MRIs can thus either unexpectedly reveal or confirm the presence of (suspected) arachnoid cysts. Of further diagnostic impor-tance is the fact that, in most cases, arachnoid cysts are congenital. Less commonly, arachnoid cysts may develop due to head injury, tumor, infection or brain surgery. Regardless of the cause, these cysts can be either asymptomatic or symptomatic.

Given this background information, consider the following (fictional) case:

A 20 year old female snowboarder with no significant previous health history sustains a concussion after a fall on the mountain. The diagnosis of concussion is made clinically and no imaging studies are performed at the time of diagnosis. However, the woman presents to the clinic one year later describing intermittent headache (which is sometimes severe enough to cause vomiting) as well as visual disturbance. An MRI performed at this time reveals the presence of an arachnoid cyst.

Although the patient's symptoms started almost immediately after the concussion, and thus it seems likely that the concussion is their cause, what is not clear in this case is whether or not the patient's symptoms are related in any way to the arachnoid cyst. Notice that this particular uncertainty is unrelated to the accuracy of the MRI. Even if the MRI is an accurate representation of the situation in the patient (i.e., even if the cyst is "really" there and not some sort of imaging artifact), the uncertainty remains because the patient had no baseline MRI prior to the concussion, nor did she receive one at the time the concussion was diagnosed. Thus it would not be possible for the team to determine whether either.

(a) the fall caused the arachnoid cyst
or
(b) the fall potentially exacerbated a previously present arachnoid cyst

In other words, even if the MRI is accurate in this case, the diagnosis is still uncertain as it is not clear whether or not the patient's symptoms are due to the presence of the cyst. Yet, the answer to this question matters: if the cyst is causing the symptoms then it will need to be treated, either by open craniotomy and fenestration or by extracranial shunting. Both of these procedures carry a significant medical risk, but they also both carry a significant potential benefit: *if* the cyst is the cause of the patient's symptoms, then removing it will relieve the patient of the symptoms. On the other hand, if the presence of the cyst is unrelated to the patient's symptoms, then either of these treatment procedures would be a waste of time and resources and would also be too risky for the patient to undergo.

3.5   Medical Imaging

In the above example, we have assumed that the MRI is an accurate representation of the state of affairs in the patient's brain. However, in many cases of medical imaging additional epistemic uncertainty arises because medical images are not simply photographs:

In contrast, the format of data from functional neuroimaging experiments is not originally in the format of an image, but rather in terms of data structures that encode numerical values of phase and frequency-dependent signal intensity collected in an abstract framework called "k-space". Visual representations of data in k-space bear no visual resemblance to images of brains. These data are transformed to spatial values of signal intensity with a Fourier transform, resulting in an image that looks roughly brain-like. This analytical transformation doesn't alter the information encoded in the data, and thus may be taken not to introduce any inferential distance, in that it introduces no error or range of possible causes. However, the radical transformations in format are indication of the indirectness of the technique relative to photography. The fact that these transformations are completely invisible to the consumer of the image implies that neuroimages are not revelatory, and illustrates the inaptness of the imposition of an epistemic framework paradigmatic of photography. (p. 25).

What this "inferential distance" means is that, "ambiguities and lack of complete data, and physical limitations such as diffraction, field non-uniformity and so on, prevent the image from being an exact representation of what would be seen if the imaged part of the patient were to be exposed to direct vision or drawn by an artist" (Sarvazyan et al. 1991).

Indirect representation or "inferential distance" and the question of accuracy is not a problem specific to medical imaging. In fact, most (if not all) scientific models whether in physics, biology, chemistry or economics, can be understood as indirect representations of their target systems as well. The question that we most often want to answer when it comes to scientific (or medical) models or images is: how do these indirect representations provide good -or at least adequate- explanations of the target systems that they represent? Or, in the medical context specifically, how can medical images, which are incomplete representations, lead to an accurate diagnosis?

In the philosophy of science literature, attempts to answer the question of how scientific models explain have generally centered on first analyzing the concept of representation, since it is usually assumed that scientific models explain because they represent their target systems. But although many philosophers of science agree that scientific representation is important for model explanations, what exactly representation amounts to has been the subject of much debate. Very generally, traditional accounts of scientific representation can be divided into two groups: what I will call "strong" accounts and "weak" accounts. Although these two types of accounts are presented as alternatives to one another in the literature, both rest on a common understanding that there is either a formal or an informal relationship of similarity between a model and the target system that it represents and that this relationship is the basis of the model's explanatory power. Strong accounts of scientific representation say that there is a shared underlying mathematical or mechanistic structure between a model and a target system that comprises the representational relationship between the two. "Weak" accounts of scientific representation, on the other hand, argue that the model-target relation is something weaker than partial isomorphism. In many cases, scientific models explain via comparison cases (Kennedy 2012; Jebeile and Kennedy 2016). Arguably, this is also often the way medical images work in a diagnostic context. That is, when working towards a diagnosis, physicians often mentally compare a medical image with a mental image of the relevant patient body part reconstructed from "a knowledge base of anatomy, pathology, histology, physical properties of tissues etc" (Sarvazyan et al. 1991). If the medical image is different from the mental image, this information can then be used as evidence towards a diagnosis of disease or disorder. But of course we are interested in making correct diagnoses in medicine, so one might well ask whether or not the image displayed on the monitor accurately represents the reality in the patient in question (Chhem 2010). This is not a simple question to answer as: the black and white image obtained is conventionally "displayed" as a variation of tissue densities (CT), signal intensities (MRI) or echogenicity (ultrasound). To make this "scientific image" to closer resemble the actual [body part], computer programs enable the manipulations of cross-sectional 2-d images into a volumetric image. This is "post-processing," i.e., processing after the data set was acquired. The result is a "3-d reconstruction" of the 2-d images (Chhem 2010).

In other words, the image is clearly an artificially created one, and we are left with the question of what is "the link between the patient's body part and the image displayed on the monitor?" Whether we understand this link to be a "strong" one of isomorphism or a "weak" one of similarity, we are still left with the question of when or whether the MRI or CT images in question "provide sufficient information to achieve a diagnosis" (Chhem 2010).

Medical images alone, as we can see from the case study above, are never enough for an accurate diagnosis, no matter how accurate a representation it is. Instead, the medical image, because it is a form of indirect observation, must be interpreted in the clinical context, and this requires an appeal to other forms of evidence. In other words, although the epistemic situation of diagnostic uncertainty in many instances cannot be avoided completely, it is still possible to approach it strategically in order to avoid (or at least mitigate) negative outcomes for both patients and physicians. Some of these potential negative outcomes that can arise from mismanaged diagnostic uncertainty in the clinical setting include the epistemic (in the form of overdiagnosis or underdiagnosis), the pragmatic (in the form of increased financial and time costs), and the ethical (in the form of increased patient suffering). More specifically, both overdiagnosis and underdiagnosis can increase clinical costs as well as patient suffering, and thus we should aim to avoid them whenever possible. One way to do this is to properly interpret diagnostic imaging tests in the clinical context.

3.6   Analysis

This case is representative of many others like it both because of the diagnostic uncertainty inherent in it and because of the fact that the medical team will be required to act even in spite of this. Diagnostic uncertainty is often present in medical imaging cases like this one because, epistemically, medical images, as we have seen, are indirect representations of what is occurring in the patient, and also because "advanced imaging studies show tremendous details of pathology. [But] they can also show incidental findings that are of unclear significance" (https://www.aafp.org/afp/2014/1201/p784.html). What this means practically is that while diagnostic images can accurately reveal masses, lesions and other structures, these images alone do not a diagnosis make. Instead, diagnostic images must be interpreted – and this interpretation must take place in the context of other clinical evidence. This is true of all diagnostic tests, not just of imaging studies: in order for the result of a diagnostic test to have any meaning in a clinical context, that result must be given an interpretation. Again, this is the case independent of test or imaging accuracy. Simply having an accurate test result does not automatically give us an accurate diagnosis:

In other words, [determining] whether or not a given diagnostic test is accurate is not exactly like asking whether or not a given tape measure is accurate. In the case of a tape measure, all we need to do is compare the tape measure with some reference standard, such as the standard metre in Paris, in order to determine whether or not it is accurate. But in order to determine whether or not a given diagnostic test yields accurate diagnoses [...] we need to understand how to interpret the quantities [or images] that the test measures [or reveals]. (Kennedy 2016).

This means that all diagnostic test results must be interpreted in the clinical setting, otherwise they will not have any meaning for either the patient or the practitioner.

In this particular case, there is an extra layer of uncertainty regarding the interpretation of the MRI result because of the lack of a baseline study. In fact, one might worry whether imaging studies should even be performed in cases like this, if the medical team will question the results of the diagnostic study, no matter what it reveals. The answer to this question is not a simple one, but the short version of the answer is that the diagnostic process in cases like this is actually not much different than the process in cases in which baseline studies *are* available. In both types of case, the diagnosis will depend both on what the imaging study shows and on the clinical context. If the imaging study reveals a dramatic finding then more weight should be given to the consideration of its diagnostic significance. Similarly, when patient symptoms are severe, even modest imaging findings can be of significant clinical importance.

Perhaps this answer seems obvious. However, it contains an implicit critique of the evidence based medicine paradigm. Evidence based medicine (EBM) has been the dominant paradigm in clinical medicine since the 1990s. And while the movement has been applauded for moving away from the old style of paternalistic medicine that privileged a physician's clinical experience above all else, it has also been criticized for its over-reliance on statistical studies, as well as on diagnostic images and tests. Recently, some have argued that we should be pluralists when it comes to what counts as medical evidence. For example, Clarke et al. (2014) have argued that both statistical and mechanistic evidence are required in order to establish a causal claim (about treatment effectiveness) in medicine. I am sympathetic to this view and here I will extend it further, beyond treatment considerations, to diagnosis. In my view, while diagnostic studies, images and tests are indeed valuable evidence toward a diagnosis, they are only one sort of evidence, not the only sort, and case studies, mechanistic reasoning, patient interviews and even physical exams should also be counted as evidence toward a diagnosis as well. Indeed, evidence other than diagnostic test evidence is often required in order to make an accurate diagnosis in a given patient case. Again, this is because even when diagnostic studies give us accurate information, this information is meaningless unless it is given an interpretation in the clinical context. Stanley (2017) makes a similar point:

Though probabilistic considerations, such as Bayesian estimations of the probability of disease given test results, are important, they are not sufficient for diagnosis selection. If these probabilistic calculations are isolated from careful observation of the particular facts of the clinical case, and if assigned prior probabilities are not tuned to clinical experience and insight, then exclusive consideration of probabilities may lead to misdiagnosis.

Further, this other evidence should not be considered to be weak, lesser or merely supportive. For instance, we know that in more than 80 percent of cases a correct diagnosis can be made based on a patient history alone (Summerton 2008), and that if "the history and physical examination are linked properly by the physician's reasoning capabilities, laboratory tests should in large measure be confirmatory" (Campbell and Lynn 1990). In addition, mechanistic reasoning can help to confirm a suspected diagnosis, and many consider a good (or "gold standard" diagnosis to be one that proposes a causal explanation, for two important reasons. First, knowing the cause of a patient condition facilitates treatment (by allowing for the possibility of intervening on the cause) and second, patients tend to both desire, and respond positively to, explanatory diagnoses (rather than diagnostic labels that are not explanatory) (Cournoyea and Kennedy 2014). Perhaps surprisingly, patients who understand *why* they have certain symptoms get better faster than patients who do not (Van Ravenzwaaij et al. 2010). Thus the clinical aim is generally to find a causal explanatory diagnosis for the patient's signs and symptoms. Towards this aim the ideal process of diagnosis involves taking a patient history, conducting a physical exam, and performing laboratory or imaging studies to help confirm the suspected diagnosis, while linking these components together via mechanistic causal reasoning.

If this is the ideal process of diagnosis, what does it mean in practice? Or, to put it in context, how should the medical team in our fictional case proceed? According to our previous definition of overdiagnosis, diagnosing the patient in this case with a symptomatic arachnoid cyst could potentially be wrong, in that it could be a *misdiagnosis*, but it could not be an *overdiagnosis*, since the patient is suffering from symptoms. Recall that an overdiagnosis is the diagnosis of a patient with a condition that is not currently causing the patient to suffer and will not cause the patient to suffer if left undiagnosed. Thus, on this definition, an overdiagnosis cannot occur in a symptomic (suffering) patient. Further, as long as the patient in this case is given a diagnosis of some sort, her diagnosis will not be "missed." But of course more important than classifying the type of diagnosis (or potential diagnostic mistake) in this case and others like it, is the question of how to proceed under conditions of diagnostic uncertainty. My proposal is that the best course of action in cases such as this is to engage the patient in a conversation in which the diagnostic uncertainty as well as the potential treatment options are clearly explained. In other words, diagnostic uncertainty must be communicated to the patient and not hidden. This should be done both because it is epistemically honest and because it is respectful of the patient as an active participant in the health care team. In some diagnostically uncertain cases, the best course of action may be to suspend making a diagnostic judgment. If there is truly insufficient evidence towards a particular diagnosis, and especially if the situation is not urgent, then it might be best to refrain from making a diagnosis until further evidence is gathered or an empirical trial of treatment is conducted. In other words, suspending judgment in a case does not have to result in paralysis or inaction, instead it can facilitate a treatment trial and/or further investigation.

Importantly, once the diagnostic uncertainty of a case has been communicated to the patient, the patient and the clinician or medical team should then engage in a process of shared decision-making about how to proceed. In the shared decision-making literature it is widely agreed that patients should be able to make treatment decisions that are in own their best interests – and that sharing the burden of decision-making is best for both patients and practitioners. However, the details of how this process should ideally proceed are often debated. In the case of medical imaging, while we must acknowledge that many "patients expect, and indeed want, to be informed of any potential laboratory or imaging abnormality that could possibly adversely affect their health, even if the probability that the abnormality could be injurious is highly unlikely," (https://www.aafp.org/afp/2014/1201/p784.html) in practice, clinicians are not required to give patients all available medical information, but only that information which is deemed to be medically relevant. What counts as medically relevant is of course also debated, and some have argued that "more information is always better," while others argue that too much information can overwhelm and frustrate patients. Here again, I think the best course of action is to approach informed consent and shared decision-making on a case-by-case basis. Patients who want more information are generally entitled to it. On the other hand, patients who want less information, are generally entitled to that. The key to ethical and effective communication of epistemic uncertainty in diagnosis is to carefully consider the needs of the individual patient.

3.7 Conclusion

Epistemic uncertainty regarding the interpretation of medical images can lead to overdiagnosis or underdiagnosis if not approached and managed carefully. Here I have argued that since medical images should be understood as indirect representations of the relevant part of the patient being imaged, they require interpretation in the context of other clinical evidence. Further, the clinical management of epistemic uncertainty has an ethical component: it should be honestly communicated to the patient so that the patient and clinician can move forward with diagnosis and treatment under a model of shared-decision making.

References

Broderson, John, et al. 2018. Overdiagnosis: What it is and what it isn't. *BMJ* 23: 1.
Campbell, Earl, Jr., and Christopher Lynn. 1990. The physical examination. In *Clinical methods: The history, physical, and laboratory examinations*, ed. H.K. Walker, W.D. Hall, and J.W. Hurst, 3rd ed. Boston: Butterworths.

Chhem, Rethy. 2010. Medical image: Imaging or imagining? In *Medical imaging and philosophy*, ed. Heiner Fangerau, Rethy Chhem, Irmagard Muller, and Shih-Chang Wang. Dordrecht: Springer.

Clarke, Brendan, Donald Gillies, Phyllis Illari, Federica Russo, and Jon Williamson. 2014. Mechanisms and the evidence hierarchy. *Topoi* 33 (2): 339–360.

Cournoyea, Michael, and Ashley Kennedy. 2014. Causal explanatory pluralism and medically unexplained physical symptoms. *Journal of Evaluation in Clinical Practice* 20 (6): 928–933.

Hofmann, Bjorn. 2017. The overdiagnosis of what? On the relationship between the concepts of overdiagnosis, disease, and diagnosis. *Med Health Care and Philos* 20: 453–464.

Jebeile, Julie, and Ashley Kennedy. 2016. Explaining with models: The role of idealizations. *International Studies in the Philosophy of Science* 29 (4): 383–392.

Kennedy, Ashley. 2012. A non representationalist view of model explanation. *Studies in History and Philosophy of Science* 43 (2): 233–420.

———. 2016. Evaluating diagnostic tests. *Journal of Evaluation in Clinical Practice* 22: 575–579.

Rogers, Wendy, and Yishai Mintzker. 2016. Getting clearer on overdiagnosis. *Journal of Evaluation in Clinical Practice* 22: 580–587.

Sarvazyan, A.P., et al. 1991. A new philosophy of medical imaging. *Medical Hypotheses* 36 (4): 327–335.

Stanley, D. 2017. The logic of medical diagnosis: Generating and selecting hypotheses. *Topoi* 38 (2): 437–446.

Summerton, Nick. 2008. The medical history as a diagnostic technology. *British Journal of General Practice* 58 (549): 273–276.

Van Ravenzwaaij, J., T.C. Olde Hartman, H. Van Ravesteijn, R. Eveleigh, E. Van Rijswijk, and P.L.B.J. Lucassen. 2010. Explanatory models of medically unexplained symptoms: A qualitative analysis of the literature. *Mental Health in Family Medicine* 7: 223–231.

Chapter 4
Screening, Scale and Certainty

Stephen John

Abstract A common concern about screening programmes is that there is much uncertainty about their effects. Using the example of CT-based screening for lung cancer, this paper explores the sources of uncertainty and possible strategies for reducing uncertainty. Specifically, it suggests that there is an epistemologically and ethically significant distinction between "individual-level" and "population-level" uncertainties, such that reducing uncertainty in the interpretation of images may not reduce the uncertainties which are most practically relevant.

Keywords Screening · Uncertainty · Lung cancer · Image interpretation

4.1 Introduction

Lung cancer is a significant cause of morbidity and mortality in much of the developed world; for example, it is the third most common cancer in the UK (46,700 new cases per year), accounting for 21% of all cancer deaths (Cancer Research UK 2019). Since at least the 1920s, there has been widespread consensus that the earlier that cancers are detected and treated, then the more effective treatment will be (Lowy 2011, Chap.3). This consensus underlies screening programmes, which aim at the early detection of cancers in asymptomatic individuals. Unsurprisingly, there has been much interest in the possibility of introducing screening programmes for lung cancer. Of course, details vary across different studies, but the basic idea is simple: screening programmes identify a population deemed to be at "high risk" of lung cancer, who are then invited to a low-dose CT scan. Radiologists study this scan to see if they can detect any unusual masses ("nodules"); if nodules are detected, then subsequent follow-ups, decided on the basis of their size and volume, are used to determine whether they are cancerous. A large-scale study in the US was widely

S. John (✉)
Department of History and Philosophy of Science, University of Cambridge, Cambridge, UK
e-mail: sdj22@cam.ac.uk

© The Author(s), under exclusive license to Springer Nature Switzerland AG 2020
E. Lalumera, S. Fanti (eds.), *Philosophy of Advanced Medical Imaging*, SpringerBriefs in Ethics, https://doi.org/10.1007/978-3-030-61412-6_4

reported as showing that low-dose CT-based screening can have significant impacts, most notably a 20% reduction in lung-cancer related mortality compared to screening with x-rays (National Lung Screening Trial Research Team 2011). However, this study – and other, similar studies – have been met with a large degree of scepticism (Henaghan 2019). First, there are debates over whether these studies have, in fact, shown the "gains" they claim to have shown (Gigerenzer 2015). Second, there are debates over whether these studies have adequately captured the "costs" associated with screening. Two sources of "costs" are particularly relevant to this paper: first, there are costs associated with "false positives", that is to say, incorrectly identifying benign growths as cancerous growths); second, there are costs associated with "overdiagnosis", that is to say, treating cancerous growths which would not have gone on to cause significant symptoms had they been left untreated (Brodersen et al. 2017). (Note that there is a further concern in many cases: that screening modalities may themselves cause harm. As CT scans tend to involve a much lower dose of radiation than x-rays, I place these concerns to one side here).

Imagine, then, that you are a policy-maker, faced with a decision: should you institute a cancer screening programme or not? This question is difficult, because you are faced with two sorts of uncertainty. First, you face *population-level epistemic uncertainties*; i.e. given widespread disagreement, uncertainty in establishing what the effects of the programmes will be. Second, even were these uncertainties resolved you might face *population-level ethical uncertainty*; i.e. uncertainty as to whether the "benefits" of the programme – say, number of lives saved – ethically outweigh the "costs" – say, of number of cases of overdiagnosis. To make matters worse, it seems that these uncertainties are inter-related: if you think that not enacting an effective programme would be a significant ethical error, then this might influence your tolerance for epistemic uncertainty (Douglas 2009).

We typically think that good policy should be based on good evidence. Uncertainty about our evidence and what it shows seems, then, to undermine policy-making. Fortunately, there may seem to be a simple way in which to reduce both ethical and epistemic uncertainties around lung cancer screening: by reducing the uncertainty in the screening encounters. To explain: one of the key challenges in screening programmes is that many of the results of screening tests are, themselves, of uncertain significance; scans often reveal that patients have very many nodules in their lungs, few of which are (pre-)cancers. It seems plausible that, were we to find strategies for reducing or mitigating these *individual-level* uncertainties (i.e. uncertainties about the significance of specific findings in specific individuals), then we could also reduce both population-level epistemic uncertainties and population-level ethical uncertainties. In turn, such a thought may – at least in part – underlie moves towards AI-assisted screening in domains such as lung cancer screening, where such technologies are touted not only on the grounds of reduced cost, but increased reliability (Ross 2019). Particularly when combined with hype about the development of AI, the simple thought that reducing individual-level uncertainty will help reduce (both forms of) population-level uncertainty is seductive. But is it true?

This chapter raises a series of worries about the simple thought. Specifically, it is structured around four questions:

- What, precisely, does it mean to reduce the uncertainties in the screening encounter?
- Which epistemic strategies might best reduce those uncertainties?
- Will resolving these uncertainties help with the epistemological question?
- Will resolving these uncertainties help with the ethical question?

My broader aim in addressing these questions is to clarify the relationships between the interpretation of medical images, knowledge of the underlying mechanisms of disease, and broader population-level knowledge and concerns. I seek to understand the relationships, both epistemological and ethical, between individual-level and population-level perspectives. After addressing each of my questions (in Sects. 4.1, 4.2, 4.3, and 4.4 respectively), I return to this general theme in the Conclusion.

4.2 Reducing Uncertainty in Interpreting Images

What does it mean to reduce the uncertainties inherent in the screening encounter? To address this question, consider a (slightly stylised) example, based on a recent UK study into the viability of routine low-dose CT screening (Field et al. 2016). Imagine a radiologist who is sent a scan: she sees something which looks like a nodule. She must now decide which of four categories the nodule sits in. She decides that it meets the criteria for being a category 3 nodule, "larger, probably malignant". In-line with the national protocol, she recommends a 3 month check-up.

Of course, identifying a category 3 nodule may save a patient's life. This is a weighty benefit. On the other hand, lung cancer screening, testing, and treatments can cause substantial harms (Bach et al. 2012). To simplify a hugely complex topic, let us just assume that if that nodule is, in fact, a (precursor to a) cancer which will go on to cause symptoms, then receiving this result will, ultimately, be in the patient's best interests. However, if it is not, then receiving this result will not be in the patient's interests: rather, she will, at best, have three months of unnecessary worry before getting the all clear (i.e. the finding is a "false positive"), and, at worst, might end up having surgery for a cancerous growth which would not, in fact, have harmed her anyway (i.e. she will be a victim of overdiagnosis and overtreatment). There are many questions we can ask about the radiologist's judgment. However, given the ultimate goal of medicine is to help, rather than harm, patients, the most pertinent question is simple: how likely is it that the patient will benefit from the radiologist's claim that "this is a category 3 nodule"?

Very broadly, we can distinguish four kinds or sources of uncertainty relevant to answering this question.

First, the radiologist may be uncertain whether the image on the scan is a nodule *at all*. Although CT scans are improving, making an image of the inside of human lungs is no simple matter. In interpreting images of the lungs, it can be difficult to distinguish between nodules and other aspects of the internal architecture. Typically, this fact is posed as a problem for assessing radiologists' sensitivity: i.e. there are worries that they may fail to identify nodules at all. However, there is also good evidence that trained radiographers and radiologists can interpret images as representing nodules when, in fact, they are not (Rubin 2015). Estimates of the rate of such findings vary widely, and, presumably, turn both of the available technology and on idiosyncratic features of the individual radiologist.

Second, even if the radiologist is correct that the image is one of a nodule, she may be uncertain in her judgment that this nodule is a Category 3 nodule. Although the criteria for being a Category 3 nodule are highly precise – "if solid and intraparenchymal, a volume of 50–500mm3. If solid and pleural or juxtapleural, a diameter 5–9.9mm. If non-solid or part solid, a diameter of the ground-glass component of >5mm. If part solid, the solid component has a volume of 15–500mm3 or a maximum diameter of 3.0–9.9mm" – establishing that some detected nodule meets these criteria is no simple or mechanical task. In studies, there is often disagreement between radiologists and radiographers over the correct categorisation of nodules (Field et al. 2016). Even though radiologists are, in general, slightly better at nodule categorisation, these discrepancies give any individual radiographer good reason to question her categorisation, particularly when measurements are near the operational margins. Unfortunately, nature does not require that nodules present in ways which are easy to measure or assess.

Third, even if the radiographer is correct that this is a category 3 nodule, she may be uncertain that this nodule will, in fact, turn out to be cancerous at all. This is, in fact, surprisingly common: for example, in the recent UK study, out of 472 cases of "category 3 cancers", nine patients ended up being treated for lung cancer. This is not necessarily to imply that the judgment that these growths fell into "category 3" was incorrect: rather, the uncertainty stems from the fact that nodules can be in category 3, but harmless. Remember that, according to standard classifications, a category 3 nodule is "*probably* malignant"; i.e. it might very well not be cancerous at all.

Fourth, even if the radiographer is correct that the nodule is in category 3 and the cancer is, in fact, cancerous, it is possible that the diagnosis will be a case of overdiagnosis: i.e. that this nodule would not have progressed to cause symptoms or premature mortality in the patient's lifetime. In turn, the chances that this is true depend on several different variables: most obviously, the patient's age, but, also, the genetic makeup of this *particular* cancer, and, perhaps, evolutionary dynamics within the cancer itself (Plutynski 2018). While the first of these factors is, of course, easy to detect, the others are, in the most part, still mysteries to us. Unfortunately, while we have some evidence that the overdiagnosis rate associated with other lung cancer detection technologies is around 25%, a major meta-analysis of low-dose CT reported simply that "overdiagnosis rate for LDCT screening cannot yet be estimated" (Bach et al. 2012).

To summarise, there are at least four grounds for substantial *predictive uncertainty* over whether the (apparent) detection of a category 3 nodule will, in fact, be in the patient's best interests. Note, however, that, given the structure of the screening programme, there is an important difference between the four sources of predictive uncertainty: the first two sources involve uncertainty about *accuracy*; the latter two concern uncertainty about the *relevance* of findings.

For the first two kinds of uncertainty, there is some in-principle accessible fact-of-the-matter: whether there is a growth at all, and whether this growth meets the conditions for being a Category 3 cancer. (Note that the second fact-of-the-matter is complex, because it is only a fact relative to some way of classifying the world; still, once we have decided that the world should be classified this way, it is either true or false that a growth is in category 3 or not). In principle, it is possible to improve our ability to identify all and only category 3 growths, and, hence, reduce *uncertainty about accuracy*. (For some complexities in practice, see the next section.) For example, with more training or new machines or techniques, we might be able to become more certain both that when we say "this is a category 3 cancer", our claim is true, and that when there is a category 3 cancer, we say "this is a category 3 cancer". And, indeed, this is precisely the claim promoted by proponents of new forms of automated image recognition software (Ross 2019).

In this sense, then, we can (in principle) reduce uncertainty about whether or not our claims are "right". However, even when we are certain that we are "right" in this sense, we may still be subject to significant *uncertainty about the relevance* of being right. Even when we know that a growth is category 3, it does not follow that the growth is, in fact, cancerous: there can be "false positives". Nor does it follow from the fact that a tumour is cancerous that treatment would be in the patient's best interests ("overdiagnosis"). The first uncertainty is "built into" our ways of categorising different growths – a category 3 growth is not a *cancerous growth*, but *probably* malignant. In principle, these uncertainties can only be reduced either by changing how we classify growths or how we treat them. In turn, such changes cannot be assessed simply in terms of how well they approximate some fact-of-the-matter, because nature itself does not privilege any specific ways of classifying nodules into different categories. Rather, these categorisation schemes must be assessed, ultimately, in terms of how well they guide predictions and interventions. The second uncertainty stems from the fact that carcinogenesis is a fundamentally chancy affair (Plutynski 2018): there may, in some sense, be a fact of the matter about how a cancer would develop if left untreated, but this is not as simple or straightforward a fact of the matter as its existence, size or volume. Again, these uncertainties cannot be straightforwardly reduced other than by developing new ways of categorising cancers which more adequately predict future growth and development.

We have, then, identified two distinct sources of our predictive uncertainty. The first is uncertainty about whether we have correctly identified some image as some category of growth (uncertainty about accuracy). Even when we are certain that we do have an adequate description of the world, however, we may suffer a second form of uncertainty: uncertainty about the implications of the world being that way (uncertainty about relevance). Before turning to solutions, it is important to stress an interim conclusion. In practice, predictive uncertainty is a complex function of both sources of uncertainty: we are uncertain what to say about the likely benefits of identifying any *particular* growth, because we suffer from both *accuracy* and *relevance* uncertainty. Therefore, reducing either sort of uncertainty is an important step towards greater predictive uncertainty. However, reducing *accuracy* uncertainty is valuable only insofar as we employ useful categories for prediction. To make this point, imagine an entirely arbitrary system for classifying nodules: say, as type A (those smaller than 3.89 mm) and type B (those larger than 3.89 mm). We could develop image recognition systems which were better than any radiographer in this task, and, hence, improve imaging accuracy. However, unless we have some reason to think that the type A/type B distinction is a useful way of dividing up nodules for prediction and intervention, these gains will not translate into gains for patients. Of course, our actual systems for categorising growths are not as simple or arbitrary as my type A/type B example. Still, we should remember that getting better at measuring and classifying growths – the kinds of skills which are increasingly automated – is only one part of the challenge of reducing predictive uncertainty. We should always interrogate the value of improved accuracy by asking how, if at all, this helps the patient.

4.3   How to Reduce Uncertainty

Both accuracy and predictive uncertainty seem to stem from our inability to *see* growths as clearly as we would like: we cannot always tell the size or volume of a nodule using our technologies; we cannot see whether a nodule is cancerous or not; we cannot see the inner dynamics of cancer evolution. Therefore, it may seem that there is an obvious way of reducing uncertainty: to gain more and more knowledge at ever smaller scales. This section argues that this strategy is mistaken, with important implications for how we think about philosophy of medicine: in general, the way to reduce the uncertainties inherent in screening is to gain knowledge at the level of the population, not at the level of the cell or genome.

Accuracy uncertainty arises because images are ambiguous or difficult to understand. It may seem clear, then, that developing and investing in higher-resolution technologies will mitigate these problems (regardless of how we solve problems of *relevance*). However, while this chain of thought is appealing, it runs into a problem: as we develop higher-resolution technologies, increasingly we discover more and more growths, and are faced with more-and-more challenges in interpreting and categorising our data. Rather than discover more carcinomas we uncover more incidentalomas. As Lynette Reid has shown, if our concern is with helping patients, then cancer screening is, perhaps surprisingly, an area which bears out Wittgenstein's dictum that sometimes, an indistinct image is "exactly what we need" (Reid 2018).

What, then, is an effective strategy to reduce uncertainty about accuracy? We can represent the problem of accuracy in Bayesian terms: the effect of an "observation" of a category 3 cancer on our credence that the individual in question has a category 3 cancer does – or should – turn on the background likelihood that the individual has a category 3 cancer in the first place (i.e. the base rate of disease). This basic logical point implies a simple strategy for reducing accuracy uncertainty: by narrowing the population we screen, such that we screen only those who are already more likely to have cancer. The higher the base rate of cancer in the population, then the more certainty we gain from a positive test result. Indeed, this is part of the basic logic of screening programmes; such programmes do not necessarily screen the entire population, but, rather, "at risk" populations. (Note, for example, that even the impressive US NLST results – of a 20% decrease in lung-cancer mortality – involved a trial focussed on heavy smokers; we would expect far less impressive results within a wider population). The best way of identifying "at risk" groups is through the use of population-level statistics, which establish strong correlations between certain demographic features and cancer-related outcomes. For example, various studies have sought to establish risk factors for lung cancer, with the aim of constructing risk-models which allow us to stratify the population according to risk. Using these risk scores to narrow the screened population does not change anything in the radiologist's judgment of the images in front of her – unlike, say, introducing higher-definition screening tools – but it does reduce the uncertainty inherent in translating clinical judgment into patient relative predictions.

I will now turn to uncertainties about relevance. As I explained above, even when we are certain that some growth does fall into some category, we may still face significant uncertainty about whether that growth is cancerous, and, if so, the likely path of carcinogenesis. In turn, this uncertainty is particularly problematic from patients' perspective, because it can lead to overdiagnosis and, hence, overtreatment. Plausibly, these uncertainties stem from the fact that cancerous growths – even growths of the same organ-of-origin – display a wide degree of genetic heterogeneity, such that some grow far faster and more virulently than others (Plutynski 2018). In turn, recognition of this heterogeneity has stemmed new developments in pharmacogenomic medicine, with attempts to tailor treatments to specific cancer sub-types, characterised in genomic term (Berry 2015). It may seem, then, that a similar strategy should pay dividends in cancer screening and early detection contexts: through diligent study of genomic = level differences in cancer, and related differences in their cellular-level effects, we might be able to construct more specific ways of categorising nodules which would, in turn, allow us to make more precise predictions (for an extreme version of this hope, see Lange 2007).

However, while there is some truth to the thought that greater genomic- and cellular-level knowledge might help us construct better schemes for categorising cancerous growths, this strategy faces significant challenges. Given the inherent complexity of biological systems (Mitchell 2009) translating increased knowledge of the cellular-level effects of different genomic mutations into usable schemes for categorising growths is no simple task. Furthermore, at least in the short term, there is a far simpler strategy we might use for reforming our classification schemes: by running large-scale, population-level studies investigating whether alternative categorisation schemes reduce the rate of overdiagnosis. For example, we can, at least in principle, compare different ways of categorising screen-detected growths on overall disease-specific mortality, and use this knowledge to identify schemes which allow us to make more accurate, patient-relevant predictions.

I have suggested that the most effective routes to reduce screening uncertainties are likely to rely on *via* population-level epidemiological studies. This suggests an important disjunction between the *ontological* causes of uncertainty and the best *epistemic strategies* for reducing uncertainty. Much of our uncertainty stems from the difficulty of identifying and characterising cancers at a *micro*-scale, but the best strategies for overcoming these uncertainties seem to involve moving to the *macro*-scale. One feature of this move to the macro-scale is that, to a very large extent, we can simply eschew all talk of causation: it does not matter whether the demographic traits we use to identify high-risk groups track actual *causes* of cancer, as opposed to mere *correlates*, because we use these features solely to reduce our uncertainty, rather than as themselves tools for intervention. There is here, then, a larger moral for recent work in the philosophy of medicine, where many commentators have developed an influential argument from Russo and Williamson (2007) that the population-level knowledge generated by the tools of Evidence Based Medicine must be supplemented by mechanistic knowledge. Such claims may have some clout if we are using studies to infer *causal* claims, but they do not necessarily hold true when we are using population-level studies for *prediction*.

Before moving on, it is important to note a further problem. In thinking about reducing uncertainty, we sometimes face trade-offs. First, there may be trade-offs between reducing *accuracy* and *relevance* uncertainty. While a more complex scheme for categorising early growths may, in principle, do a better job at reducing false positive rates (say), this scheme is useful only insofar as it can be operationalised. A system for categorising early growths into 20 subtypes might in a perfect world reduce *relevance* uncertainty, but it's not much use in the actual world if we are awful at *accurately* classifying growths in this way. Second, within various practices, there may be trade-offs between different sorts of errors: for example, some new categorisation scheme may decrease our chance of "false positives", but only at the cost of increasing our chance of "false negatives" or reduce the chance of over-treatment at the cost of increasing the chance of undertreatment. In such cases of "epistemic risk", we may have to make a choice about which kinds of epistemic error we think are more important to avoid (Douglas 2009). Plausibly, no amount of factual knowledge will resolve these questions. Instead, they must be settled by distinctively practical – prudential, ethical or political concerns. I return to these issues in more detail in Sect. 4.4 below.

4.4 Does It Help? 1: Resolving Population-Level Uncertainty

The previous two sections have outlined some of the sources of patient-relevant uncertainty in interpreting radiological images, and suggested how these problems may be overcome through use of population-level data. However, the key motivating question behind this paper is whether reducing such patient-relevant uncertainty will also reduce the population-level uncertainties faced by policy-makers, who must decide whether to institute cancer screening problems. As the Introduction explained, policy-makers face two kinds of uncertainty: epistemic uncertainty about the likely outcomes of a screening programme; and ethical uncertainty about whether these outcomes are morally acceptable. This section considers the first kind of uncertainty: will reducing individual-level uncertainty take the heat out of the screening wars?

We can distinguish two broadly factual questions a policy-maker must ask about some programme: what will its likely effects be?; how much will it cost? (In the language of health policy: How effective is the programme? How cost-effective is it?) I will focus on the first. There are huge disputes over the likely effects of instituting lung cancer screening programmes. Broadly, we can distinguish two kinds of worries. The first concerns the quality and interpretation of completed studies. For example, there are on-going debates over whether studies showing a decrease in Disease Specific Mortality imply a concomitant decrease in All Cause Mortality (Henaghan 2019); it can be difficult to calculate the overdiagnosis rate associated with screening; and it can be hard to disentangle the effects of screening from other causes of mortality decline. A second set of debates arises even when study results are uncontroversial: whether we can safely extrapolate from the fact that an intervention worked *there* that it will also work *here* (Cartwright 2012). For example, it is possible to think that the US National Lung Screening Trial (2011) did show a significant decrease in lung cancer related mortality, but doubt that this implies that a similar drop would be seen from introducing a similar programme in the UK, because of background differences between the national contexts (for example, in the provision of healthcare or the base-rate incidence of lung cancer).

On the face of it, reducing individual-level uncertainty should have an impact on population-level uncertainty: the better we can predict the benefits and harms for each affected individual, then the better we can predict population-level outcomes. However, there are three reasons to think that reducing individual-level uncertainty will be the best or most effective way in which to reduce population-level uncertainty.

First, a high degree of individual-level uncertainty is compatible with a high-degree of population-level certainty. For example, it is possible that we might be able to infer the likely population-level overdiagnosis rates associated with some screening programme with a high degree of certainty – for example, on the basis of large-scale epidemiological studies – while remaining entirely uncertain about the likelihood that any specific individual will be over-diagnosed (i.e. our knowledge of individual-level heterogeneity may block us from equating each individual's chances of overdiagnosis with the population average). Therefore, reducing individual-level uncertainty is not necessary for reducing population-level uncertainty.

Second, even if reducing individual-level uncertainty can reduce *some* population-level uncertainty, it is not sufficient for eradicating it. There are many more sources of population-level uncertainty about the effects of programmes than the uncertainties inherent in the screening encounter. For example, predicted changes in the lung cancer rate – say, as a result of changes in smoking behaviour – may make it hard to predict the likely future population-level effects of a programme, even if that programme is highly effective at identifying genuinely dangerous growths. Further, introducing a screening programme may have further effects on individual behaviours, and, hence, population-level health outcomes, regardless of the accuracy of individual-level predictions. For example, making smokers aware of their increased risk of lung cancer may, itself, prompt healthy behaviour change (indeed, a common theme in the literature on lung cancer screening is that the encounter offers an opportunity to promote smoking cessation).

Third, and most importantly, reducing uncertainty in the interpretation of images may not tell policy-makers what they most want to know. Consider one of the core debates in the screening wars: whether we should measure the effects of screening in terms of Disease Specific Mortality or in terms of Overall Mortality. Often, cancer screening programmes seem to show a decrease in Disease Specific Mortality but no corresponding decrease in Overall Mortality. Proponents of screening seek to explain away this apparent discrepancy, claiming that studies are simply too small to detect the (real) effect on OM. Opponents of screening, by contrast, provide an alternative explanation, that unchanged OM measures are evidence of the hidden costs of screening: roughly, that even if screening programmes are saving lives lost to specific cancer sub-types, they are also causing significant harms – for example, through exposure to radiation or unnecessary, risky treatment. These debates are important because policy-makers should care about the *overall* effects of screening policies, rather than their effects on cancer-related mortality *per se*; if screening's proponents are correct, then, when implemented at a sufficiently large scale, reductions in DSM will translate into reductions in OM; if opponents are right, then screening programmes will have no – or even a negative – impact on OM. (For a useful overview of these issues, see Bach et al. 2012).

These debates around the proper interpretation of population-level studies are relevant to the links between individual-level uncertainty and population-level uncertainty. Imagine that, through the strategies outlined in the previous section, we become better-and-better at identifying all and only those growths which would, if left untreated, cause symptoms or premature mortality. This reduction in individual-level *predictive uncertainty* should, in principle, allow us to become more-and-more certain about the likely *population-level* effects of screening on cancer-related morbidity and mortality. However, this greater degree of individual predictive certainty will not tell us anything about the likely effects of screening on *overall* mortality, because it will not tell us anything about the likely costs of screening, subsequent testing and treatment on those for whom, ultimately, screening (and subsequent rounds of testing) were unnecessary. Through refinement of screened populations, we might become more certain that those we screen and treat will be benefited by our interventions, but this is still compatible with very many people being exposed to ultimately unnecessary invasive medical procedures. In turn, knowing the extent and magnitude of these costs is central to making an informed judgment of the overall consequences of screening. Greater individual-level certainty may help us get a better grip on the population-level benefits of screening, but not on its population level costs.

Reducing individual-level predictive uncertainty will often help to clarify some aspects of policy-relevant, population-level uncertainty. However, we should not think that all of the concerns and questions relevant to policy-making can be resolved this way. Consider, again, proposals to replace human radiographers with image recognition software. Imagine, for the sake of argument, that we could show that using these automated techniques would improve screening accuracy. This knowledge may make it slightly less difficult to figure out the likely population-wide effects of a screening policy; it doesn't, however, make it easy.

4.5 Does It Help? 2: Resolving Ethical Uncertainty

Even if we could predict the overall pattern of effects of a proposed screening programme, this knowledge does not suffice to make a decision about whether to pursue it. Rather, we also need some way of assessing whether those effects are, all-things-considered, ethically valuable. This is no easy task because it involves at least two steps: first, we need to commensurate these outcomes so as to allow us to compare them along a single scale (for example, to translate mortality and morbidity effects into effects on QALYs); second, we need some principle to tell us when a particular pattern of benefits and harms is choice-worthy. Both of these steps are controversial: should we use QALYs or DALYs? Should we care only about the net effects of a policy or, also, about whether it reduces health inequalities? (Hausman 2015). And these controversies are heated, at least in part, because they involve contested ethical value judgments: for example, about the relationship between health and well-being, or about the correct account of the demands of justice. Even a policy-maker who is certain about the effects of a screening programme may be very uncertain as to whether those effects are, all-things-considered, good or bad. (And, even if she is *herself* morally certain, democratic norms may require her to take account of moral disagreement, and, hence, act *as if* she is uncertain (Schroeder 2017).)

Will greater individual-level certainty help the policy-maker resolve her ethical uncertainty? On one level to ask this question is to make a philosophical mistake: assuming a fact/value distinction, no set of factual claims can ever resolve ultimate ethical disagreements. At a more practical level, however, factual knowledge can resolve ethical tensions, because it can help us to realise that we were wrong that a certain choice does, in fact, involve some value conflict, or it can help us identify routes out of a dilemma. For example, when faced with an inescapable ethical dilemma – say, between saving one life and saving many people from a lesser fate – my dilemma may be resolved if I learn that saving the one is, in fact, impossible, or if I learn that there is some way in which to save both the one and the many. Similarly, we might think that if we create new screening programmes where individual-level uncertainty is reduced, then some of the ethical tensions around screening will be resolved or reduced. Rather than be forced to choose between, say, promoting net population health and reducing health inequalities, we might be able to identify policies which both promote health and reduce inequalities. Clearly, something like this is possible. Unfortunately, I suggest that greater individual-level certainty is, if anything, likely to exacerbate, rather than to reduce, ethical dilemmas about screening.

Screening policy seems to raise two key ethical tensions. The first is a tension between different ethical principles concerning outcomes. On the one hand, we might think that, in medical contexts at least, we should never choose policies whose outcomes include the imposition of medically unnecessary harms (i.e. we should be bound by non-maleficence); on the other, we might think that we should always choose outcomes which do as much good as possible (i.e. we should be bound by beneficence) (Childress and Beauchamp 2001). In screening, these principles seem to pull in opposite directions: we know that the best way in which to do as much good as possible is to screen as many people as possible; but we also know that the more people we screen, then the more likely it is that we will cause unnecessary medical harm through overdiagnosis and overtreatment. Will greater individual-level predictive certainty help resolve this tension? No. As Sect. 4.2 explained, we best gain greater individual-level predictive certainty by narrowing the population we screen; this policy would reduce the risks of overdiagnosis, and, hence, seem in line with the principle of non-maleficence. However, reducing the number of people we screen has a cost in terms of promoting as much good as possible, because screening "low" or "moderate" risk populations is a highly effective way of catching as many cases of cancer as possible. This is a simple corollary of what Rose called the "fundamental axiom of preventive medicine": that "a large number of people exposed to a small risk may generate many more cases than a small number of people exposed to a high risk" (Rose 2008, 59).

The second key ethical uncertainty in screening concerns the relationship between *ex-ante* and *ex-post* ethical perspectives. This tension also stems from Rose's fundamental axiom: if we want to save as many lives as possible, then, plausibly, the best strategy is to focus on "moderate risk", rather than "high risk" populations. However, quite apart from non-maleficence concerns, such policies seem in tension with a plausible ethical principle that we should pay more ethical attention to those at greatest risk of harm (John 2014). To make this tension vivid, consider a stylised example: many seem to think that it is more valuable to reduce a 0.5 risk of death imposed on 10 people in the population than a 0.01 risk imposed on 1000 people, even if we can reasonably expect that the latter policy would save more lives overall (Daniels 2012). This tension between a concern for the *ex-ante* distribution of risk and a concern for maximising *ex-post* outcomes is one reason why screening is ethically complex. Again, gaining greater individual-level predictive certainty does not resolve, but exacerbate the tension. As noted above, the best way in which to improve individual-level predictive accuracy in screening will be to adopt programmes which more closely target interventions on high-risk individuals. In turn, these policies might be in-line with the demand that we pay greatest attention to the most at risk. However, there is also a cost to such targeted policies: if Rose is right, they are likely to have a far lesser effect on the population prevalence of disease than are population strategies. Building programmes which allow for greater individual-level certainty simply exacerbates an existing ethical uncertainty: whether we should care more about helping the most at risk or about helping the greatest number.

In short, reducing the uncertainties inherent in screening may exacerbate, rather than reduce, ethical problems around screening. Is that a bad thing? Not necessarily: it is probably preferable to discuss ethical uncertainties honestly and openly, rather than to hope that they will be cured by technological developments. Furthermore, there is something to be said in favour of hammering out our values openly: as I noted at the end of Sect. 4.2, many decisions involved in structuring a screening programme involve making trade-offs between different sorts of outcomes. We can think of these trade-offs as representing or encoding certain sorts of ethical decisions: for example, that underdiagnosis is worse than overdiagnosis. In turn, these trade-offs may play an important role in guiding screening practice: certain value judgments may, for example, implicitly guide how we categorise nodules, and these categorisation schemes, in turn, structure the process of assessing and interpreting images. Even though individual radiologists may well be unaware of this fact, their perceptions and judgments may be deeply saturated by non-epistemic values. For these judgments, then, to be proper, it seems that the values in question must be ones which are broadly justifiable to the public at large. Having a proper and full public debate over the ethics of screening may be necessary not only for the propriety of policy, but for the propriety of perception.

4.6 Conclusions

In this paper, I have discussed four, inter-related topics about the interpretation of CT-scan images in the context of lung cancer screening: why making individual-level, patient-relevant predictions on the basis of such images is so hard; how such uncertainty might be reduced; why reducing such individual-level uncertainty will not necessarily reduce population-level uncertainty about outcomes; and why reducing such uncertainty may exacerbate, rather than solve, existing ethical problems. Much more could – and should – be said about each of these topics, but my main message is simple: we cannot, and should not, detach our analysis and understanding of what does and should happen when a radiologist views some image from the broader population-level perspective. This perspective is relevant to asking the ethical question of whether someone should be making such scans and interpreting them at all; and it is central to reducing the epistemic uncertainties and ambiguities inherent in interpreting such scans. While there may be a fact of the matter as to whether or not some nodule is cancerous or not, we cannot think about the intertwined ethics and epistemology of screening without moving beyond the micro-level.

References

Bach, P., et al. 2012. Benefits and harms of CT screening for lung cancer: A systematic review. *Journal of the American Medical Association* 307 (22): 2418–2429.

Childress, J.F., and T.L. Beauchamp. 2001. *Principles of biomedical ethics*. New York: Oxford University Press.

Berry, Donald A. 2015. The brave new world of clinical cancer research: Adaptive biomarker-driven trials integrating clinical practice with clinical research. *Molecular Oncology* 9 (5): 951–959.

Brodersen, C., et al. 2017. Overdiagnosis: What it is and what it isn't. *BMJ Evidence Based Medicine* 23 (1): 1.

Cancer research UK. 2019. *Lung cancer statistics*. https://www.cancerresearchuk.org/health-professional/cancer-statistics/statistics-by-cancer-type/lung-cancer. Accessed 09 July 2019.

Cartwright, N. 2012. Presidential address: Will this policy work for you? Predicting effectiveness better: How philosophy helps. *Philosophy of Science* 79 (5): 973–989.

Daniels, N. 2012. Reasonable disagreement about identifed vs. statistical victims. *Hastings Center Report* 42 (1): 35–45.

Douglas, H. 2009. *Science, policy and the value-free ideal*. Pittsburgh: University of Pittsburgh Press.

Field, J., et al. 2016. The UK Lung Cancer Screening Trial: A pilot randomised controlled trial of low-dose computed tomography screening for the early detection of lung cancer. *Health Technology Assessment* 20 (40): 1–146.

Gigerenzer, G. 2015. Five year survival rates can mislead. *British Medical Journal 2013* f548: 346.

Hausman, D.M. 2015. *Valuing health: Well-being, freedom, and suffering*. Oxford: Oxford University Press.

Henaghan, C. 2019. Understanding lung cancer screening. *BMJ EBM Blog*. https://blogs.bmj.com/bmjebmspotlight/2019/02/15/understanding-lung-cancer-screening/.

John, S. 2014. Risk, contractualism and Rose's prevention paradox. *Social Theory and Practice* 40 (1): 28–50.

Lange, M. 2007. The end of diseases. *Philosophical Topics* 35 (1/2): 265–292.

Lowy, I. 2011. *A woman's disease: The history of cervical cancer*. Oxford: Oxford University Press.

Mitchell, S.D. 2009. *Unsimple truths: Science, complexity, and policy*. Chicago: University of Chicago Press.

National Lung Screening Trial Research Team. 2011. Reduced lung-cancer mortality with low-dose computed tomographic screening. *New England Journal of Medicine* 365 (5): 395–409.

Plutynski, A. 2018. *Explaining cancer*. Oxford: Oxford University Press.

Reid, L. 2018. Is an indistinct picture "exactly what we need"? Objectivity, accuracy, and harm in imaging for cancer. *Journal of Evaluation in Clinical Practice* 24 (5): 1055–1064.

Rose, G. 2008. *The strategy of preventive medicine*. Oxford: Oxford University Press.

Ross, C. 2019. Google's AI improves accuracy of lung cancer diagnosis, study shows. *Stat News* May 29th, 2019. https://www.statnews.com/2019/05/20/googles-ai-improves-accuracy-of-lung-cancer-diagnosis-study-shows/.

Rubin, G. 2015. Lung nodule and cancer detection in CT. *Journal of Thoraic Imaging* 30 (2): 130.

Russo, F., and J. Williamson. 2007. Interpreting causality in the health sciences. *International Studies in the Philosophy of Science* 21: 157–170.

Schroeder, S.A. 2017. Using democratic values in science: An objection and (partial) response. *Philosophy of Science* 84 (5): 1044–1054.

Part II
Social Epistemology

Chapter 5
On the Inclusion of Specialists as Authors in Systematic Reviews

Rodney J. Hicks, Lauren J. Hicks, and Robert E. Ware

Abstract Although advocated by some methodologists involved in the procees of evidence-based medicine and consequent health technology assessment, we argue that exclusion of content-area experts from systematic review teams would represent a massive detriment to clinical knowledge formulation and ultimately patient care. We believe that arguments in favour of this suggestion are both intuitively flawed and unsupported by direct high-level evidence that patients will benefit. In our opinion, the evidence and argument that is advanced in support of this thesis lacks intellectual rigour and is demonstrably unbalanced. We contend that fundametal principles of fairness must assume that doctors generally hold the best interests of their patients to be paramount in their considerations, that patients have the right to assuming that experts are engaged in the formulation of evidence that potentially impacts their care and that professional standards are the ultimate safeguard in protecting the integrity of medical opinion.

Keywords HTA · Systematic reviews · EBM · Professionalism · Methodology

R. J. Hicks (✉)
Cancer Imaging, Peter MacCallum Cancer Centre, Melbourne, VIC, Australia

The Sir Peter MacCallum Department of Oncology, The University of Melbourne, Melbourne, VIC, Australia
e-mail: rod.hicks@petermac.org

L. J. Hicks
Mercy Hospital for Women, Heidelberg, VIC, Australia

R. E. Ware
Cancer Imaging, Peter MacCallum Cancer Centre, Melbourne, VIC, Australia
e-mail: rob.ware@petermac.org

© The Author(s), under exclusive license to Springer Nature Switzerland AG 2020
E. Lalumera, S. Fanti (eds.), *Philosophy of Advanced Medical Imaging*, SpringerBriefs in Ethics, https://doi.org/10.1007/978-3-030-61412-6_5

57

"All sciences are vain and full of errors that are not born of experience, the mother of all knowledge." Leonardo da Vinci

5.1 Introduction

Strategies to minimize bias in the collection, analysis and interpretation of data have been progressively implemented in medical research over several decades. Input from statisticians, epidemiologists and clinicians has refined clinical trial design and informed peer-review processes within the medical literature as well as guiding secondary analyses within the domain of health-technology assessment (HTA). These methodologies have been particularly utilized in the creation of the knowledge base that has supported access to new imaging technologies, such as positron emission tomography (PET), but are also applicable to broader aspects of medical practice.

Despite the generally cooperative nature of the collaboration between the stakeholders and their mutual motivation to enhance patient care, as in many aspects of human interaction, there has been competition for pre-eminence in the field of evidence-based medicine (EBM). In support of their own claims to priority, "methodologists" can argue that clinicians are irrevocably subject to self-interest as providers of healthcare services and therefore can't be trusted to provide unbiased guidance to either patients or policy-makers. Clinicians, conversely, can equally question whether patients are better-off relying on knowledge formulated by individuals or groups with neither specific expertise related to their particular condition, nor practical experience in clinical care. Emphasizing the importance of experience, they echo Da Vinci's view of science.

Clinicians face a critical point in the history of medicine at which their role as "experts" is increasingly being diminished and their integrity in acting in the best interests of their patients is often disputed. For example, eminent figures in the EBM field have quite recently recommended that, by default, teams performing systematic reviews and meta-analyses should exclude content-area experts, defined as specialist clinicians and authors of original research in the area under review, from authorship (Gøtzsche and Ioannidis 2012). In their opinion, experience in caring for real-world patients would seem to count for little and to add nothing beyond the prospect of making systematic review manuscripts more interesting to clinicians themselves. There are several reasons why this proposal demands careful philosophical consideration by the medical community and bioethicists. These include the presumption of innocence, the right to self-determination and the concept of professionalism.

5.2   The Presumption of Innocence

The proposal that practical expertise needs to be purged from the process of legiti-mising medical knowledge depends on the view that content-area experts have an unhealthy propensity to obscure the truth through personal bias. The theory goes that content experts are intolerably captive to self-interest as well as lacking the necessary analytical skills to judge the merits of medical evidence. Existing guide-lines mandating an authorship role for specialist clinicians are dismissed as harm-ful – the *"taming"* of evidence-based medicine (EBM) by *"the centuries old, expert based power system in healthcare"*(Gotzsche and Ioannidis 2012).

This thesis leaves inescapable questions unstated and unanswered. How could specialist clinicians be trusted to put patients' interests first in clinical-care deci-sions if they are, by default, too compromised by self-interest to even contribute to judgements about what constitutes gold-standard medical knowledge? How could content-experts be trusted to conduct primary scientific research, without which meta-analyses and systematic reviews would be impossible? Should clinical medi-cine devolve to algorithms developed solely by "methodologists" – statisticians, epidemiologists, heath economists and others with little or no experience in super-vising the care of real-world patients?

One could take a Freudian view that by virtue of their training, experiences and contact with like-minded individuals, clinicians become incapable of recognizing unconscious patterning of opinion and motivation to protect themselves and are, thus, largely powerless to change. Alternatively, one could adopt an Adlerian per-spective that clinicians are entirely capable of self-reflection, personal change and motivation to be valuable to others by virtue of the altruism that is a traditional ethos of the medical profession. The concept that clinicians are incapable of recognizing and dealing with their own biases for the greater good of society denies them of the presumption of innocence in regard to their behaviour within the confines of EBM or HTA.

We fully agree that clinicians have ample opportunity to put their own interests first, and some clinicians do take unfair advantage of their power and privilege. Further, we concede that some content-area experts do not do enough to minimize bias in the primary research, reviews and editorials they are responsible for. Yet overreacting to these limitations will not help patients achieve better outcomes.

5.3   The Right to Self-Determination

Clearly, the primary focus of EBM should be the patient and their right to determine the best course of investigation or treatment for their possible disease process. Would patients seriously consider not having the input of expert clinicians into management decisions in their individual case? Enthusiasm to remove clinical expertise from systematic review teams disrespects the importance of the doctor-patient relationship and the trust required on both sides for effective decision-making.

The primacy of patients in EBM has been repeatedly emphasized by Sackett and fellow founders of this methodology. In their seminal paper- "Evidence based medicine: what it is and what it isn't"- they stipulated that doctors practising evidence-based medicine *"will identify and apply the most efficacious interventions to maximise the quality and quantity of life for individual patients."* These authors recognised that clinical expertise is entirely relevant to the process of incorporating patient preferences into a management strategy that fits their individual needs. The authors were unambiguous in their view that increasing clinical expertise is reflected by *"more thoughtful identification and compassionate use of individual patients' predicaments, rights, and preferences in making clinical decisions about their care"* (Sackett et al. 1996) and that *"without clinical expertise practice risks becoming tyrannised by evidence, for even excellent external evidence may be inapplicable to or inappropriate for an individual patient."* Further they cautioned that external evidence *"can inform, but can never replace, individual clinical expertise."*

Apparently dismayed at the failure to adequately communicate the crucial interplay between the elements of EBM, Sackett subsequently commented in a letter that *"we clinicians who accept the awful responsibility of caring for individual patients with their unique risks, responsiveness, values and expectations have simply failed to communicate key elements of our decision-making to some ethicists and methodologists who don't diagnose and treat individual patients...their [ethicists and methodologist's] definition of evidence-based health care stops with external evidence and ignores the other 2 of its 3 vital elements: clinical expertise and patients, values"* (Sackett 2000). Further, Gotzsche wrote in his 2007 book, *"Rational Diagnosis and Treatment"* (Gøtzsche and Wulff 2007), that good clinical research *"can only be carried out by experienced clinicians".*

Could methodologists gain sufficient understanding of clinical context simply by referring to textbooks or review articles, notwithstanding the irony that these sources of knowledge are written by the very content-area experts that some contend are untrustworthy? The thesis in question is also silent about the paucity of direct high-level evidence showing secondary data-analyses do actually improve patient-important outcomes. This is surprising given that a leading methodologist has documented multiple ways for meta-analyses to introduce bias and lead to conflicting and even erroneous conclusions (Ioannidis 2010). Furthermore, no mention is made of the limited potential for secondary analysis to improve estimates of truth compared to the primary data itself (Egger et al. 2001). Highly-respected methodologists recognise that the main benefit of systematic review and meta-analysis is to gain an understanding of the reasons for disparate conclusions of primary studies, editorials and "non-systematic" reviews (Egger et al. 1997). Content-experts have first-hand perspective on the clinical relevance of the research data so surely incorporating content-experts may circumvent errors born of inexperience rather than threatening "truth".

As access to medical information becomes more available to patients through the internet, patient autonomy or shared decision-making is increasingly paramount in respect to self-determination in healthcare. Accordingly, it must be questioned whether patients would, or should, trust information that deliberately excludes input from expert clinicians. To allow them this choice, any such information should be clearly identified as such in order not to mislead patients as to the source of opinions reached.

This also applies to the evaluation of new technologies through the process of HTA. Increasingly, analyses of available evidence to support, or deny, reimbursement are commissioned by government or other sources of healthcare funding, including private health-insurers. With a clear focus on limiting government expenditure or maximizing profit in the private-sector, combined with intrinsic risk-aversion, these bodies generally have a bias against funding new technologies. Organisations with the expertise and manpower to perform the literature reviews that are needed within HTA are often highly dependent on the funding provided by these bodies and are therefore, themselves, faced with a conflict-of-interest. For example, IQWiG, which evaluates new medical procedures in Germany, is exclusively commissioned by the Federal Joint Committee of the Federal Ministry of Health and is financed through levies derived from statutory health insurance funds (https://www.iqwig.de/en/about-us/responsibilities-and-objectives-of-iqwig/contracting-agencies-and-funding.2951.html). While it states that *"no interest group can influence the results of reports produced by the Institute"*, this inter-reliance between government agencies and insurers, and the purveyors of HTA evidence gathering, could potentially bias its conclusions. It is interesting to note that the reports of IGWiG on positron emission tomography (PET) have consistently failed to endorse the use of this modality in conditions in which it has been approved in other jurisdictions and is recommended in clinical guidelines published by professional bodies that, themselves, derive no direct benefit from provision of healthcare services.

Our own experience of the HTA process has demonstrated the potential for political influence to negatively impact the results of EBM reviews and restrict or delay patients' access to a new technology (Ware 2004; Ware et al. 2004). Systematic reviews published following a process of HTA are badged as the highest level of evidence and stated to reflect the opinions of experts conscripted into the review. If the views of these experts were to be ignored or misrepresented, patients could be potentially misled in their personal decisions in accessing these technologies, whether reimbursed or not.

The Australian experience of clinical experts having their names and associated scientific credibility misrepresented for political purposes is not unique. A 1996 report on Positron Emission Tomography generated in the United States incorporated an appendix with the names of several clinical experts involved in an *"Advisory Committee to the PET Assessment"*. Personal communication with two of the experts listed, Steven Larson and James Fletcher, suggested that their contribution to the scientific validity of this report was misstated. Responding to the question, *"Were your comments fairly represented in the final document?"*, Larson wrote, *"As I recall, our expert medical opinion was not given much weight, in comparison to the opinion of health technology experts who believed strongly in the concept of evidence-based medicine as a guide to practice." He continued, "The review was tilted in favor of a negative conclusion by setting up criteria for study design after the fact...I have thought of this experience since as science in the service of a political agenda- namely, the VA administration was not anxious to spend money on PET imaging, but did not wish to appear reluctant to improve the health care of the veteran with lung cancer".* Balancing the conflicting interests of financing healthcare and delivering quality healthcare argues for the advocacy of clinicians in representing the interests of patients, particularly when the goal of the process is to determine whether reimbursement is provided or not. Supporting these views, James Fletcher wrote, *"I believe there was an over-arching agenda and a political motive for the study that would allow the VA to continue to have a moratorium on the purchase of PET scanners based on the results of this study".* (Personal communications 2003).

Certainly, we are aware of no high-level, direct evidence showing that excluding content-area experts from secondary data-aggregation processes results in a closer approximation of the truth.

5.4   The Concept of Professionalism

The tenet that content-area experts allow personal interest to subvert the truth is a strong element of the recommendation that they should be excluded from the preparation of systematic reviews and, presumably, HTA. Apparently a *"flurry of reviews, editorials and letters from content area experts that try to refute, or even denigrate"* are published when *"convincing randomized controlled trials or systematic reviews find results that invalidate expert based practice"*. However, some evidence presented to back this claim concerned a widely-disputed meta-analysis of screening mammography (Gotzsche and Olsen 2000) and closer examination reveals that some vociferous published criticism came from methodologists, not just content-experts (Moss et al. 2000; Nystrom 2000; Hayes et al. 2000). The process of scientific advancement through the ages has relied on disputation and challenging of dogma. The peer-reviewed literature has long benefitted from commentaries and rebuttals of errors, perceived or proven. It is through this process that knowledge approaches but can never fully achieve truth.

Similarly, published commentary on the COURAGE trial (Teo et al. 2009) also supposedly shows that content-area experts, in their fervour to defend lucrative expert-sanctioned practice, ignored high-level evidence that percutaneous coronary intervention (PCI) *"didn't work"* in stable coronary artery disease. However, symptomatic relief of medically refractory angina is the accepted clinical indication for undertaking PCI, and both the systematic review (Katritsis and Ioannidis 2005) and the COURAGE trial showed that angina was substantially reduced after PCI when compared to medical therapy. With a reasonable clinical perspective, inability to show statistically significant improvements in the "hard" endpoint of all-cause mortality is neither surprising nor particularly relevant to patients who are selected for PCI according to expert-derived practice guidelines. Who could argue that amelioration of debilitating symptoms following PCI in an eighty-year-old patient with severe medically refractory angina constitutes evidence of an invalid expert-based practice?

"Not everything that counts can be counted, and not everything that can be counted counts." **(From a sign hanging in Albert Einstein's office)**

Are patients safe in the hands of methodologists blinkered by their belief that what really counts are statistically-precise mean values for easily measured outcome measures? The penchant of methodologists to attribute great value to questions of little consequence to real patients reminds us of the tongue in cheek proposal to conduct a double blind RCT to assess the value of parachutes for preventing "gravitational challenge" injury (Smith and Pell 2003). Sadly, this humorous attempt to draw attention to the misplaced focus of methodologists does not appear to have resulted in commensurate restraint.

Our recent experience in the field of cancer imaging further emphasizes the material danger of judging clinical scientific research within a vacuum of inexperience.

For some years, respected methodologists have pushed the view that reliable diagnosis is passé – at best a surrogate indicator of patient benefit. Recently this counterintuitive stance has hardened to a new orthodoxy asserting that *"true-negative patients"* must be studied in randomized controlled trials to determine whether *"decreasing the intensity of treatment is actually accompanied by an improvement in patient-relevant outcomes"*(Scheibler et al. 2012). Taken to its logical extension, this could involve randomising people who had cancer excluded on imaging to receiving or not receiving chemotherapy and assessing whether avoiding chemotherapy improved patient outcomes. The suggestion of exposing people who don't have disease to demonstrably harmful interventions violates a primary ethical value – *primum non nocere* (first do no harm). We are alarmed that influential methodologists could first voice, and then seek to defend, unethical concepts of clinical research and patient care (Hicks et al. 2012, 2013).

In her book, *"Dark Age Ahead"*, Jane Jacobs foresees the loss of self-regulation by the learned professions as a tipping point for society. To suggest that the professional ethics that have guided medicine for centuries, that have put the interests of the patient foremost in the minds of doctors and that have been the focus of altruistic self-sacrifice cannot be relied-on in the fundamental process of review of evidence is to deny the concept of professionalism.

Even if we accept the tenet that some clinicians fail to achieve a fair balance between their own and patients' interests, is there less reason to suspect that some methodologists may also be subject to bias? Our own experience suggests that this is not the case. We have, for example, documented how methodologists, funded recurrently by governments to perform literature reviews, are responsible for bias that compromised the scientific integrity of systematic reviews of positron emission tomography (PET) scanning (Hicks et al. 2012; Ware and Hicks 2011). Intentional omission of data from relevant primary studies and factual errors in reporting original data and authors' conclusions contributed to the adoption of clinically inappropriate decision-making benchmarks. In Australia, there is proof that a "systematic review" of PET that has strongly influenced cancer care for more than a decade was conducted to meet the government's hidden expenditure limit, with substantial evidence that evaluation of scientific data was prejudiced from the outset. Ultimately, a purportedly independent scientific evidence review was completely perverted by Australian Government "editorial" intervention (Milne 2008), given the "primary finding" of "insufficient evidence" of clinical effectiveness was added to draft reports by government officials who also watered down the clinicians' true findings to provide "logical consistency" in the altered report. As a result of a Senate Committee Enquiry, one of the authors of this manuscript (RJH) was granted leave to have his name removed from those alleged to have supported the validity of this review.

Given direct evidence that methodologists may engage in unscientific and potentially illegal practices that obscure truth and ultimately prejudice patient outcomes, we think it unwise to accept a thesis that also overplays the failings of content-area experts. It is gratifying that some methodologists do openly recognise that they are well-positioned to derive personal benefit from their roles as pre-eminent judges of evidence (Schunemann et al. 2008).

The role of government is also pertinent to any consideration of competing interests. Although much attention is devoted to drug companies clouding the truth for the sake of corporate profits, in most countries governments are much bigger players in their healthcare systems. Governments have a vested interest in making voters believe that their healthcare budgets are equitable, economically rational and evidence-based. Could anyone suggest that there is no possible relationship between rapidly expanding government funding for methodologist groups whose systematic review can be promoted as gold-standard knowledge, the commensurate rise in career prospects for methodologists, and enthusiasm for excluding content-area experts who can spoil the party by invoking their practical experience in looking after real-world patients?

There is already evidence that the involvement of imaging specialists in systematic reviews is declining. Sardanelli et al. reviewed over 800 systematic reviews of imaging procedures performed over a decade and found that only 38% involved a radiologist or nuclear medicine specialist but that those that did had a significantly and statistically higher quality rating (Sardanelli et al. 2014).

5.5   Conclusion

Exclusion of content-area experts from systematic review teams would represent a massive detriment to clinical knowledge formulation and ultimately patient care. We believe that arguments in favour of this suggestion are both intuitively flawed and unsupported by direct high-level evidence that patients will benefit. In our opinion, the evidence and argument that is advanced in support of this thesis lacks intellectual rigour and is demonstrably unbalanced.

Ultimately, the imperfections in clinical-research methodology and application of its result to the care of individual patients are unavoidable but we must not make rash decisions in our quest to minimise errors and uncertainty. In our view, individual patients will best be served if broad clinical questions are addressed by bringing different perspectives and skills to bear on problems, much in the manner that multidisciplinary meetings address difficult individual management decisions. Expertise is maximised, the possibility of base instincts prevailing is minimised and, to some extent, monitored.

One thing is clear to us. There is no sense attempting to address the ever-present potential for error in clinical knowledge formulation by eliminating the input of people who have practical and comprehensive experience of what really matters to patients in favour people who do not.

Contributors and Sources   The authors have expertise in internal medicine with 2 (RJH and REW) being specialists in nuclear medicine and one (LJH) having expertise in biostatistics. All contributed to the writing and review of the paper.

Competing Interests   All authors have completed the ICMJE uniform disclosure form at www.icmje.org/coi_disclosure.pdf (available on request from the corresponding author) and declare: no support from any organisation for the submitted work; no financial relationships with any organisations that might have an interest in the submitted work in the previous three years; and no other relationships or activities that could appear to have influenced the submitted work.

References

Egger, M., G.D. Smith, and A.N. Phillips. 1997. Meta-analysis: Principles and procedures. *BMJ* 315 (7121): 1533–1537.

Egger, Matthias, George Davey Smith, and Douglas G. Altman. 2001. In *Systematic reviews in health care: Meta-analysis in context*, ed. Matthias Egger, George Davey Smith, and Douglas G. Altman, 2nd ed. London: BMJ Books. (2003 [printing]).

Gotzsche, P.C., and J.P. Ioannidis. 2012. Content area experts as authors: Helpful or harmful for systematic reviews and meta-analyses? *BMJ* 345: e7031. https://doi.org/10.1136/bmj.e7031.

Gotzsche, P.C., and O. Olsen. 2000. Is screening for breast cancer with mammography justifiable? *Lancet* 355 (9198): 129–134. https://doi.org/10.1016/S0140-6736(99)06065-1.

Gøtzsche, Peter C., and Henrik R. Wulff. 2007. *Rational diagnosis and treatment : Evidence-based clinical decision-making*. 4th ed. Chichester/Hoboken: John Wiley & Sons.

Hayes, C., P. Fitzpatrick, L. Daly, and J. Buttimer. 2000. Screening mammography re-evaluated. *Lancet* 355 (9205): 749.; author reply 752. https://doi.org/10.1016/S0140-6736(05)72155-3.

Hicks, R.J., R.E. Ware, and M.S. Hofman. 2012. Not-so-random errors: Randomized controlled trials are not the only evidence of the value of PET. *Journal of Nuclear Medicine* 53 (11): 1820–1822.; author reply 1822-1824. https://doi.org/10.2967/jnumed.112.111351.

Hicks, R.J., M.S. Hofman, and R.E. Ware. 2013. Not-so-random errors: Randomized controlled trials are not the only evidence of the value of PET--rebuttal. *Journal of Nuclear Medicine* 54 (3): 492. https://doi.org/10.2967/jnumed.112.116020.

Ioannidis, John P.A. 2010. Meta-research: The art of getting it wrong. *Research Synthesis Methods* 1 (3–4): 169–184. https://doi.org/10.1002/jrsm.19.

Katritsis, D.G., and J.P. Ioannidis. 2005. Percutaneous coronary intervention versus conservative therapy in nonacute coronary artery disease: A meta-analysis. *Circulation* 111 (22): 2906–2912. https://doi.org/10.1161/CIRCULATIONAHA.104.521864.

Milne, C. 2008. *Matters of public interest: Positron emission tomography review in Senate Hansard*. Canberra: Senate Printing Unit.

Moss, S., R. Blanks, and M.J. Quinn. 2000. Screening mammography re-evaluated. *Lancet* 355 (9205): 748. author reply 752.

Nystrom, L. 2000. Screening mammography re-evaluated. *Lancet* 355 (9205): 748–749.; author reply 752. https://doi.org/10.1016/S0140-6736(05)72154-1.

Sackett, D.L. 2000. Equipoise, a term whose time (if it ever came) has surely gone. *CMAJ* 163 (7): 835–836.

Sackett, D.L., W.M. Rosenberg, J.A. Gray, R.B. Haynes, and W.S. Richardson. 1996. Evidence based medicine: What it is and what it isn't. *BMJ* 312 (7023): 71–72.

Sardanelli, F., H. Bashir, D. Berzaczy, G. Cannella, A. Espeland, N. Flor, T. Helbich, M. Hunink, D.E. Malone, R. Mann, C. Muzzupappa, L.J. Petersen, K. Riklund, L.M. Sconfienza, Z. Serafin, S. Spronk, J. Stoker, E.J. van Beek, D. Vorwerk, and G. Di Leo. 2014. The role of imaging specialists as authors of systematic reviews on diagnostic and interventional imaging and its impact on scientific quality: Report from the EuroAIM Evidence-based Radiology Working Group. *Radiology* 272 (2): 533–540. https://doi.org/10.1148/radiol.14131730.

Scheibler, F., P. Zumbe, I. Janssen, M. Viebahn, M. Schroer-Gunther, R. Grosselfinger, E. Hausner, S. Sauerland, and S. Lange. 2012. Randomized controlled trials on PET: A systematic review of topics, design, and quality. *Journal of Nuclear Medicine* 53 (7): 1016–1025. https://doi.org/10.2967/jnumed.111.101089.

Schunemann, H.J., A.D. Oxman, J. Brozek, P. Glasziou, R. Jaeschke, G.E. Vist, J.W. Williams Jr., R. Kunz, J. Craig, V.M. Montori, P. Bossuyt, and G.H. Guyatt. 2008. Grading quality of evidence and strength of recommendations for diagnostic tests and strategies. *BMJ* 336 (7653): 1106–1110. https://doi.org/10.1136/bmj.39500.677199.AE.

Smith, G.C., and J.P. Pell. 2003. Parachute use to prevent death and major trauma related to gravitational challenge: Systematic review of randomised controlled trials. *BMJ* 327 (7429): 1459–1461. https://doi.org/10.1136/bmj.327.7429.1459.

Teo, K.K., S.P. Sedlis, W.E. Boden, R.A. O'Rourke, D.J. Maron, P.M. Hartigan, M. Dada, V. Gupta, J.A. Spertus, W.J. Kostuk, D.S. Berman, L.J. Shaw, B.R. Chaitman, G.B. Mancini, W.S. Weintraub, and Courage Trial Investigators. 2009. Optimal medical therapy with or without percutaneous coronary intervention in older patients with stable coronary disease: A pre-specified subset analysis of the COURAGE (Clinical Outcomes Utilizing Revascularization and Aggressive druG Evaluation) trial. *Journal of the American College of Cardiology* 54 (14): 1303–1308. https://doi.org/10.1016/j.jacc.2009.07.013.

Ware, R. 2004. Health technology assessment (HTA) groups have been instrumental in restricting patient access to PET worldwide. *Journal of Nuclear Medicine* 45 (12): 1977.

Ware, R.E., and R.J. Hicks. 2011. Doing more harm than good? Do systematic reviews of PET by health technology assessment agencies provide an appraisal of the evidence that is closer to the truth than the primary data supporting its use? *Journal of Nuclear Medicine* 52 (Suppl 2): 64S–73S. https://doi.org/10.2967/jnumed.110.086611.

Ware, R.E., H.W. Francis, and K.E. Read. 2004. The Australian government's review of positron emission tomography: Evidence-based policy-making in action. *The Medical Journal of Australia* 180 (12): 627–632.

Chapter 6
Development of Novel Radiopharmaceuticals: Problems, Decisions and More Problems

John W. Babich and Uwe Haberkorn

Abstract The development of new tumor targeting radiopharmaceuticals also named tracers relies on the identification and validation of new target structures or processes in close conjunction with the application of new techniques for the development of new biocompatible molecules. A radiopharmaceutical/tracer consists of a carrier molecule which transports the tracer to the target and the radioactive isotope which allows visualization and/or therapy. These techniques either use known lead structures for further refinement or try to identify new lead compounds which is then followed by the screening of various derivatives of these molecules. Their further evaluation and optimization consist in the characterization of the structure-function relationships and subsequent improvement with respect to binding, internalization and biodistribution by rational design of corresponding analogues. However, during this process several decisions have to be made with regard to the nature of the disease process which should give some hints for useful targets, the method for identification of the target and the choice to follow or skip a project. This is usually based on reasonable choices based on the evidence available to minimize the risk for failure. Sometimes this may result in selection without preferences.

J. W. Babich
Division of Radiopharmaceutical Sciences and MI3 Institute, Department of Radiology, Weill Cornell Medicine, New York, NY, USA

Citigroup Biomedical Imaging Center, Weill Cornell Medicine, New York, NY, USA

Sandra and Edward Meyer Cancer Center, Weill Cornell Medicine, New York, NY, USA

U. Haberkorn (✉)
Department of Nuclear Medicine, University Hospital Heidelberg, Heidelberg, Germany

Clinical Cooperation Unit Nuclear Medicine, German Cancer Research Center (DKFZ), Heidelberg, Germany

Translational Lung Research Center Heidelberg (TLRC), German Center for Lung Research (DZL), Heidelberg, Germany
e-mail: uwe.haberkorn@med.uni-heidelberg.de

Keywords Radiopharmaceuticals · Tracers · Nuclear medicine · Research · Drug development · Uncertainty

'I had a dream that I was awake and I woke up to find myself asleep.' Stan Laurel

6.1 Introduction

New molecules create future opportunities for nuclear medicine diagnostics and therapeutics. The implementation of novel molecular entities into clinical practice requires a line of research and development which relates scientific findings to knowledge of pharmacology, radiochemistry and finally medical needs. We should be aware that there are important differences between the design and development of pharmaceuticals and radiopharmaceuticals. First, for radiopharmaceuticals only radioactivity matters not the amount of the carrier molecule as there is no chemically induced pharmacological effect. In essence, the 'effect' is the radioactivity. The quantity of a tracer given to the patient is very low, i.e. a sub-pharmacological dose, whereas a pharmaceutical by definition has to be given at a pharmacologically effective dose. Second, the target for a radiopharmaceutical must not necessarily be causally involved in the development of disease. It may just be linked or associated with the disease phenotype (a feature such as a unique protein expression) or the status (e.g., rate of growth or metabolic activity) of the disease. Proteins controlling cellular homeostasis may not be the best choice as a target because the difference between normal function and the diseased state may be only modest. This means that often slight differences in the equilibrium of intracellular processes are causing disease. However, without a significant differential between states diagnostic or therapeutic radiopharmaceuticals are unlikely to find utility. Furthermore, intracellular targets are more difficult to address than targets which are located at the extracellular site of the cancer cell membrane, because for intracellular targets the radiopharmaceutical has to pass the membrane first. Basically, the key question is: how can we direct as much radioactivity as possible to a tumor and for a sufficient period of time to allow a radioactive atom to deposit its energy in a manner sufficient to kill or visualize cancer cells. Simultaneously, we need this phenomenon to be absent in normal tissues! Therefore, carrier molecules that specifically bind to and transport radionuclides to the tumor which present minimal or reduced normal tissue affinity/interaction are a unique necessity of radiopharmaceuticals.

During the last years we also have learned that cancer cells may not be the only cells that represent or possess attractive potential targets within the mass of a tumor, but within this mass are also protein and cellular components of tumor stroma and the tumor microenvironment. This means also that non-tumor cells and matricellular proteins, proteins which are located in the extracellular space, can represent potential targets some of which are highly unique to tumors. In essence, in our fight to rid a patient of a malignancy we can target cancers (malignant cells) or tumors (the complex mass including malignant cells).

The process of tracer development can be described as a chain of consecutive steps starting with defining the clinical need. What follows then is identifying a target closely associated with the clinical problem, followed by target validation, identification of molecular entities capable of binding to the target, creation and identification of possible structural leads (chemicals with known target binding), synthesis and in vitro screening of an array of related structures (to improve binding), and subsequent conversion (radiosynthesis) of screen hits to radioactive molecules for an iterative evaluation of in vitro and in vivo biological characteristics and behaviors (potencies).

The outcome of this process can reveal many problems related to the initial hypothesis (targeted), choice of methodology (capability of synthetic approaches and adequacy of screening models) and interpretation of the resulting data. Commonly, the in vitro and in vivo validation effort results in disqualification of many ligands or the realization of the need to modulate the choice of the starting lead structure to achieve enhanced affinity and/or stability.

Finally, an initial proof of concept study may be done in patients (Haberkorn et al. 2017). As we know this step is full of risks. The pharmaceutical industry invests large amounts of capital to generate data from both preclinical (animal) experiments and clinical (human) trials. In spite of these efforts, less than 14% of projects that initiate clinical trials end up being registered as drugs (Wong et al. 2018). The lowest probability of success in clinical development is in Phase II, when drugs are tested for efficacy (Wong et al. 2018). This high failure rate is partly reflective of the complexity and variability of human physiology, which increases the cost of successful therapies. Of note, the overall probability of success for oncology is the lowest at 3.4%. Although clinical trials with biomarkers enabling patient selection at various stages of investigation do substantially better, it results in a meagre doubling of the probability (Wong et al. 2018).

6.2   Choice of a Target: A Crucial Decision

First of all we have to ask whether it is really necessary to develop a drug that targets a single process (protein) with very high affinity or might it be better to hit multiple targets with a cocktail of agents? The proposal to use a cocktail of targeting tracers immediately begs the question: since multiple targets may be expressed in multiple normal organs and, as a consequence, the drug may accumulate in these normal organs, will we increase the number of side effects? For diagnostic applications of radiopharmaceuticals the corollary would be: is there an increased background with a lower contrast? However, there are at least examples showing that low-affinity multi-target drugs such as NMDA receptor agonists have a reduced range of side-effects (Lipton 2004; Rogawski 2000). This may be different for radiopharmaceuticals because in that case side affects are not expected anyway, but still an increase in background activity in nuclear medicine imaging may occur. With respect to therapeutic applications of radiopharmaceuticals this may result in an unfavorable dose to normal organs, thereby, narrowing the therapeutic window.

The second question is related to the efficacy. It is believed that a high affinity molecule binding strongly to one specific target is more effective in neutralizing this target and/or its related pathways. However, a weak linkage of a drug to its receptor does not necessarily mean that it has no effects. Many proteins involved in the intracellular signaling or transcription processes have a weak binding to each other (Rogawski 2000). Because of this fact and bearing in mind that we mostly face networks of interactions it is possible that even a drug with weak affinity might achieve a significant influence on the network. This is based on two assumptions:

1. the mechanism which has to be subjected to treatment can be interpreted as a network
2. in order to guarantee the function of the mechanism the elements of the network have to interact

The network approach has been used for example for the identification of a protein function e.g. by comparing transcriptional networks from different organisms (Stuart et al. 2003; Bergmann et al. 2004) or by the determination of protein-protein interactions (Archakov et al. 2003) and in studies dedicated to a metabolic control analysis (Cascante et al. 2002). However, the usual procedure in drug development in pharmaceutical industry consists of finding a target with a pathologically associated function, identify a high affinity ligand by screening random or tailored libraries or by rational design, make proof-of principle experiments and engage in clinical applications. This approach favors high affinity binders rather than low affinity agents.

However, several highly efficient drugs such as NSAIDs, salicylate, metformin or Gleevec are different: they target many targets simultaneously. In addition, therapies of complex diseases such as cancer or infections are more frequently planned as combinations giving up the one drug-one target principle. Another example are plants which use various factors to respond to pathogenic threat. According to Csermely et al. this shows that using multiple molecules is an evolutionary success story (Csermely et al. 2005).

Multiple partial attacks inside of a network may be more efficient than the complete knockout of a single component (target) of this network (Agoston et al. 2005). This is thought to be due to the fact that partial multiple interactions are able to block a higher number of nodes in the network than a single knockout (Agoston et al. 2005). In addition, usually multi-target drugs have a lower affinity which makes the druggability easier and, therefore, increases the size of the druggable proteome (Korcsmaros et al. 2007). If one supposes a sort of generality of network behavior in biology (Csermely 2004; Watts and Strogatz 1998) then there may be many multi-target drugs available. This has been exemplified by Modos et al. (2017). Using a systems level approach of the protein networks in colon, breast, liver and lung cancer they investigated the influence of first and second neighbors of cancer-related proteins such as mutated and differentially expressed proteins. This analysis revealed that mutated proteins are more central in the network than differentially expressed proteins. However, this was compensated for by a higher centrality of their first neighbors. Therefore, it seems that nodes with a central role in a network may have that role due to their interaction with their neighbors. A survey of drugs which were already on the market showed that the total number of drugs targeting these neighbors is greater than the number of drugs targeting the cancer-related proteins. Although these drugs which target the neighbors are applied mostly for non-oncological diseases, it may be possible to select some of them for a use in the setting of tumor therapy such increasing the number of druggable targets.

The concept of dual targeting with non-overlapping toxicities has been entertained in the nuclear medicine arena and seems plausible. (Bushnell et al. 2014) With respect to nuclear medicine therapies we first must recognize as has been mentioned above that the therapeutic effect arises from the delivery of ionizing radiation to the tumor and not from a pharmacological interaction of the ligand with the protein target. Where a particular molecule 'lands' can impact the effectiveness of the agent but the choice of radionuclide on the carrier molecule also defines its local 'range' of effect as within a fairly well understood radius from the point of the delivered molecule the radiation will impart its effect. The range varies based on the particle emitted with alpha particles emitting their energy within a much shorter range (50–100 microns) than beta particles (0.05–12 mm). We may ask whether therapy with a short-range alpha emitting nuclide using a single target is really the way to attack cancer if we consider that hitting multiple protein targets might have a better chance to affect the whole network than hitting one target. Since radionuclide-based approaches do not use pharmacologically relevant doses, but use the physical properties of their radionuclides, i.e. ionizing radiation as therapeutic principle, it may be questioned whether the use of alpha emitters is not inferior to beta emitters with longer range. The latter offer the hits in multiple cells and may to a certain extent compensate the heterogeneity of the target distribution in the tumor. The same may apply for the use of multi targeting tracers or cocktails of tracers addressing multiple targets. Although first evidence exists for selected applications in rare disease, it still has to be shown whether this approach is generally applicable.

Since radioactivity and its local effects are relevant and if we consider that the local effects, also of different tumor compartments, i.e. tumor cells and the constituents of the tumor stroma may lead to a network effect, i.e. multiple changes in the microenvironment, then a description of isotope-based therapy effects as a change of equilibrium within tumors makes sense.

In addition, as mentioned above, in this sense beta-emitting isotopes may be better than alpha emitting isotopes because the beta particles will cause weaker, but broader effects within the tumor network due to their physical range. Having in mind examples showing that alpha therapies sometimes work better than beta therapy we may ask whether this is a general truth. Is it just a matter of dose and beta emitters given at a dose adjusted to the difference in biological effects are equally effective at the single cell level or show even better effectiveness due to a greater network effect? It is also worth considering the role the host's immune system play in response to radiation damage to tumors and whether there is added benefit in "weaker but broader" effects that could trigger the patient's immune response in a way that recruits the host's immune cells to attack the tumor even tumor cells which are far from the local radiation (Lhuillier et al. 2019).

6.3   Target Identification and Target Validation

Target identification is performed using a variety of methods such as screening literature reports describing immunohistochemical studies, autopsy studies, genetic linkage studies, genome wide association studies, RNAi studies, proteomics, forward and reverse genetics and large-scale data sets from genomics (Lindsay 2003; Stock et al. 2015). Although constantly used by companies engaged in drug development, more and more concerns arise about the reproducibility of the reported data. This has been nicely shown in analyses by pharmaceutical companies and academia which were not able to find consistent results in the scientific reports, even when published in high-ranked journals (Stock et al. 2015; Prinz et al. 2011; Begley and Ellis 2012; Blagg and Workman 2014). This has been used as an explanation for the fact that the success rates of phase II studies dropped from 28% to 18% (Arrowsmith 2011). However, successful approaches have been reported in nuclear medicine for somatostatin receptor ligands and PSMA ligands where peptides and small molecule inhibitors have been developed as nonradioactive drugs and then used as lead structures for tracer development (Haberkorn et al. 2016). For new and less characterized targets there may be no other choice than to engage in additional studies to confirm the data presented. Since analyses in yeast and mammalian cells revealed only weak correlations of the mRNA levels with the corresponding protein levels (Pradet-Balade et al. 2001) at the end target identification has to rely on the verification at the protein level.

As mentioned above we have to ask whether it makes sense to engage in tracer development for a singular target as opposed to a multi-target approach. This largely depends on the clear description of a specific medical need and the corresponding biological/biochemical hypothesis. In order to guarantee a high accumulation of the radiopharmaceutical at the site of disease, for example tumors, several features should be fulfilled: target upregulation in the tumor tissue, a relatively large extracellular domain, absence of target shedding after ligand binding and internalization of the target-tracer complex after binding. In the optimal case all of these features are present. However, the lack of one or two of these properties may prevent development of a truly useful radiopharmaceutical.

Target validation at the protein level is usually done with immunohistochemistry (IHC) of tumors and normal organs. This method may show intra-tumoral heterogeneity which could predict treatment failure. In addition, intra-tumoral heterogeneity may also lead to sampling variability when biopsies are taken and presents a confounding factor for the validation method if IHC is made from biopsies alone (Yap et al. 2012). This phenomenon may also be responsible for the failure of the analysis of RNA expression or DNA copy number in predicting therapeutic response (Poste

2011; Sotiriou and Pusztai 2009), but it may be also be responsible for failure of targeted radiotherapy, where target-negative cells may account for non-homogeneous dose distribution within a given tumor mass leading to ensuing tumor regrowth. Besides sampling variability there is another problem concerning the use of IHC for the validation of targets suitable for the development of radiopharmaceuticals: this may be called the resolution gap. Optical microscopy works at a resolution of 0.2 μm, super resolution microscopy at 20 nm and transmission electron microscopy at 0.05 nm. In contrast the resolution of a PET scanner is at best 2–3 mm which represents a difference or gap of at least 10^4 between optical microscopy and PET. A further difference concerns the method of quantitation: semiquantitative (IHC) versus quantitative (PET). Also the molecules used for measurement are different: antibodies for IHC and antibodies, peptides or small molecules for PET. Furthermore, IHC uses tissue sections thereby underestimating processes occurring in vivo such as shedding and perfusion and clearance phenomena. These processes inevitably lead to differences in biodistribution in living subjects as compared to IHC-based pathology. In other words both methods provide a different picture of the same world and an inference from IHC to nuclear medicine procedures such as PET imaging is commonly tenuous.

Let's assume that we are able to validate several targets and IHC gives us a bundle of information showing favorable features for two or more candidates. Since drug development is a time consuming and costly endeavor we my face a situation where we have to decide which one to pursue first. How can we do that with reasonable certainty?

This may be seen as an example of a problem often discussed in philosophy. Usually the following line of reasoning exists:

1. The concept of a reasonable agent requires that a person has reasons for his actions.
2. A reasonable choice among alternatives must be based on preferences for the thing chosen among different alternatives.
3. Without preference no reason exists for a selection.

The counter-example is well known in philosophy. It is Buridan's ass staying hungry in front of two identical bundles of hay. In order not to starve the ass must choose one of these bundles. By hypothesis there is no reason to prefer one of the bundles. So either there is no reasonable choice possible in this case, or reasonable choices may exist in the absence of preference, thus attacking the above mentioned concept.

Although the example has been named as Buridan's ass, no such passage in the writings of Buridan can be found. Indeed the problem is much older as has been nicely elaborated by Nicholas Rescher (Rescher 1960). The first attempts were concerned with the place of earth in the cosmos stated by the Greek philosophers Anaximander, Plato and Aristoteles dealing rather with physical relationships. In the second step arabic thinkers such as al-Ghazal and Averroes transformed the problem to an epistemological/theological issue about the explanation of Gods choices in terms making them acceptable to human reason. The last transformation was done by the scholastic philosophers Aquinas and Buridan during ethical/theological discussions concerning human actions driven by the free will. This finally introduced the logical formulation of the paradox.

Several objections were made, mainly that such as situation does not occur in reality (Pierre Bayle 1697) or by the introduction of 'petites perceptions' which are located at a level below consciousness and drive decisions (Leibniz 1704).

A corollary of these considerations is that the case of Buridan's ass may seem to be not realistic in the real world because we may consider that situations with identical reasons for two options do not exist. Also the reasons to decide for each of the two options may be different. But it may be the case that the weight we give to each bundle of arguments for the different options is equal. This apparent equivalence is more common in practice when there are a multitude of unknowns (uncertainties that we are aware of) including the unknown unknowns (unknowns that we are not aware of) concealed within each option. In this case we also have no preference for one of the two options.

In his famous essay Rescher (1960) tried to solve the paradox with the intention to let the poor animal survive by making a choice between indiscernible hay bundles and at the same time to keep the notion of a reasonable agent. This is done by introducing a similarity between choice in the presence of symmetry of knowledge and choice in the presence of symmetry of preference. To illustrate that he introduced a similar example dealing with a person having to choose between two boxes. One containing a prize and the other being empty. Although the person has a preference for the box with the prize, he/she has a lack of information. The choice has to be made in a situation where no information is available which may guide the decision, which describes exactly the situation where there is symmetry of knowledge. Given that, the person, to act reasonable, has to find a selection without favoring one of these boxes, because there is nothing which he could use for that. That amounts to the statement that in order to avoid an artificial preference for one box, the person has to opt for a random choice. This may be done by tossing a coin or even by using a policy of choice such as selection of the alternative, which is mentioned first, i.e. a decision based on convenience. Given that, the symmetry of preference can be subsumed under the concept of symmetry of knowledge, because the available knowledge restricts the person to see the alternatives as equally desirable. Rescher concludes that the concept of random selection provides the only reasonable, because rationally defensible, solution.

Is Buridans ass now happy? And the scientist? In order to challenge the common notion that there exists a link between the number of choices and the motivation with the correlate that the ability of humans to manage and desire many choices is unlimited, Iyengar and Lepper (2000) demonstrated by three experimental settings that this is not the case. The basic concept behind these experiments was to expose the consumers to a selection between many items as opposed to a selection between a limited number of items and to quantify the number of people standing at the respective booth as well as the number of purchases. The first observation was that more people went to the booth with more items as is expected by the classical position. However, the percentage of purchases was ten-fold higher for the booth with a limited number of items. In addition, people purchasing from the booth with limited options reported a higher satisfaction with their choices. A similar observation was made when students were provided with 6 versus 30 different topics for the writing of an essay. Furthermore, the quality of the essays of the students choosing from a lower number of topics were higher than the essays from the other group. The conclusion was that, although the possibility of many choices may initially be experienced as positive and desirable, at the end it may turn out to be demotivating, a phenomenon which is coined choice overload. In this experimental situation the people placed in front of an extensive choice context enjoyed this context more, but at the same time also felt more responsible for their choice which resulted in a higher dissatisfaction and the participants were more unsure whether they made the right or the wrong decision. The more choosers see their situation as one of great complexity necessitating possibly an expert opinion the more they tend to refrain from a decision and to surrender it to another person. Unfortunately, Buridan's ass has no option to select an expert, i.e. a more sophisticated ass.

This phenomenon has been studied in detail also in three studies using functional MRI (Shenhav and Buckner 2014). The participants felt most positive, but also most anxious when choosing between products of similar high value for them. The authors found that this paradoxical experience resulted from parallel evaluations of the cost benefit ratio whereas the expected outcome tended to induce positive feelings and the consideration of the possible costs of a certain decision induced anxiety. These feelings could be tracked to the activation of different brain regions within the striatum and the medial prefrontal cortex.

It follows that we have to decide for logical as well as for psychological reasons. To do that we have to deal with uncertainty in this situation. An objective definition of the term is given by ecologists where uncertainty is characterized by a lack of information resulting in the inability to find numerical probabilities (Knight 1921; Wall et al. 2002). Alternatively, a psychological approach offers a subjective definition: uncertainty is a reaction to the external world only in the mind of the person (Head 1967). A proposal made by Hassanzadeh et al. tries to combine the objective and subjective approaches by stating that uncertainty is a subject's conscious lack of knowledge about an object which is not yet clearly defined, in a context requiring action/decision' (Hassanzadeh 2010). This definition identifies three factors of uncertainty: object, subject and context, named as uncertainty generators and is proposed to be used for solutions addressing at least the object and the context generator to obtain a reduction of uncertainty.

6.4 Leads and Ligand Libraries

Once a target is selected the hard work begins. The issues we face (in developing new radiotracers) are in some regards 'pick and shovel' approaches versus 'aspirational approaches'. We begin our trek with a review of the literature in an effort to identify a naturally occurring or previously identified ligand that specifically inter-acts with the target protein. In some cases such a ligand or substrate for the target protein is known and a crystal structure of the ligand:protein complex may be avail-able shown in great detail how this ligand 'sits' within the target protein. The latter is ideal as not only is the ligand identified but how it interacts with the protein is also known. This information can be used to create a series of compounds (compound library) that are structural derivatives of the identified/native ligand. Such a starting point may well define the best chemical or biological scaffold to use based on the structure of the 'lead' compound, i.e., antibody, peptide or small molecule. However, the search for targets does not always end with identification of a known ligand from which to start radiotracer development. In the case of identifying a high value target with no known ligand screening large libraries of random compounds may be the only way to identify a targeting molecule.

At this stage a bias is frequently introduced as we approach our target based on our compound platform of choice. A laboratory seeking to develop a radiotracer may have experience and expertise in antibody production, another in peptide syn-thesis, still another in small molecule synthesis. These three labs will each seek to approach the target using distinct classes of targeting vectors to 'answer' the same question. Without going into great detail here, these three platforms present their own advantages and disadvantages. They differ considerably in size (200–200,000 molecular weight), shape (globular, cyclic, or linear), circulation time (minutes to weeks), physiological barriers (e.g., membrane permeability, diffusion rates), excre-tion patterns, and metabolic vulnerability. They also differ in the ability to modify the vector structurally in order to tune pharmacokinetics (tissue clearance) or affin-ity (enhanced binding) for the target. While there are examples of all three platforms being used clinically for both imaging and therapy the smaller constructs (peptides and small molecules) have met with more clinical success overall. It is worth con-sidering why this is so and to understand what we know about these smaller con-structs and what we still have to learn.

It is better to know nothing than to know what ain't so. -Josh Billings

The current mindset is to knock pick and shovel and praise aspirational ventures, however much may be lost in the latter when baby and bath water are both thrown out. Small molecule and peptide approaches often require an extensive number of compounds to be synthesized and screened in order to identify subtle structural features that can define a high value lead suitable for clinical investigation. Much is learned along the way and paradigms are made, deconstructed and remade as the screening of new compounds frequently redefines the structure that leads to optimi-zation. Even after an extensive discovery effort is completed and compounds enter clinical phase of investigation the clinical results may demand heading back to the drawing board to fine tune elements of the structure. Pick & Shovel approaches lend themselves to greater understanding of the details that allow a thing to work and therefore can lead to a greater understanding of what can work in future. The 'leaps' we make are seldom seen through the lens of hard work and understanding and more through 'aspirational' hero worship. Failures are not discussed and efforts are seldom described in their entirety for various reasons. This creates a demand for a change in publication policies allowing or even demanding the publication of failing approaches.

6.5   Screening

The screening of compounds typically begins in the most artificial of ways: testing whether or not the compound binds the isolated target protein in a dish devoid of cells of bodily fluids. A cell-based assay may be a more realistic model to use for initial screening but not all putative target proteins are expressed on cell lines which can be readily obtained from commercial sources. In this case the expression has to be verified using immunohistochemistry and/or FACS (fluorescence-activated cell sorting) analysis. While molecular biology techniques allow the expression of a protein in most mammalian cells the resulting target protein-expressing cell lines may be highly artificial in terms of expression level, typical growth rate or metastatic potential compared to the disease one is attempting to recapitulate in the model. It is, therefore, important to know what the differences are between the natural occurring protein and the cells which express it and the model system used for screening. It is possible to carryout useful screening if one considers such a cell-based model as a guide to relative potencies within a group of compounds.

Transition to more biologically complex in vivo studies brings new challenges. As mentioned above, a problem which may be easily overlooked is the possibility of degradation of the target with shedding. For example, many antibodies with high affinity have been developed against mucin-1 (MUC1), but these recognized epitopes within the highly immunogenic alpha chain tandem repeat array. However, the MUC1 alpha chain is shed into the peripheral circulation, where it can complex circulating antibodies, thereby limiting their ability to reach the MUC1-overexpressing tumor cells as well as redirect radioactivity to other normal organs such as the liver and RES system (Levitin et al. 2005; Rubinstein et al. 2006). So, the critical question in this case is: what is left at the plasma membrane and can it be targeted effectively?

Another issue is the biodistribution of a putative tumor targeting drug which may result in its accumulation not only in the tumor, but also in normal tissues. This may be due to expression of the target in these normal tissues, although in lower amounts, or in unspecific accumulation by mechanisms not known a priori. Furthermore, binding to plasma proteins may prolong the circulation of the radiopharmaceutical resulting in a higher background thus leading to a lower tumor-to-background ratio. Concerning a theranostic application both, uptake in normal tissues and long circulation may lead to a higher rate of side effects when the radioactive molecules are used for treatment of cancer patients.

6.6   Interpretation

All truths are easy to understand once they are discovered; the point is to discover them.
Galileo Galilei

In its most essential form the ultimate goal of drug development is to create medicines which reduces human suffering. The path to achieve this is complex as we must first acknowledge a disease then understand its causalities or susceptibilities. Here we encounter a substantial possible error in our chosen path. There may be many causes for a disease and while diseases such as infection may have an objective causality that is ascribed to a foreign invader most other diseases may lack such a well described target. Furthermore, some pathways are shared between malignant and non-malignant diseases which is probably one of the major causes for false positive results in imaging and severe side effects in treatment. This may not be evident at the onset of tracer development. Therefore, knowledge about biological basics such as gene expression, protein relocalization, pathway activation and many other processes under varying physiological or pathophysiological conditions is needed not only at the beginning, but also during the whole sequence of drug development. In this respect data from imaging and biodistribution experiments may stimulate new basic research to clarify the role of the chosen target structure under normal and pathological conditions.

References

Agoston, V., P. Csermely, and S. Pongor. 2005. Multiple hits confuse complex systems: A genetic network as an example. *Physical Review. E, Statistical, Nonlinear, and Soft Matter Physics* 71: 051909.

Archakov, A.I., et al. 2003. Protein-protein interactions as a target for drugs in proteomics. *Proteomics* 3: 380–391. https://doi.org/10.1002/pmic.200390053.

Arrowsmith, J. 2011. Phase II failures: 2008–2010. *Nature Reviews Drug Discovery* 10: 328–332. https://doi.org/10.1038/nrd3439.

Bayle, P. 1697. *Dictionaire historique et critique.* Rotterdam: Leers.

Begley, C.G., and L.M. Ellis. 2012. Drug development: Raise standards for preclinical cancer research. *Nature* 483: 531–533. https://doi.org/10.1038/483531a.

Bergmann, S., et al. 2004. Similarities and differences in genome-wide expression data of six organisms. *PLoS Biology* 2: 85–93.

Blagg, J., and P. Workman. 2014. Chemical biology approaches to target valdation in cancer. *Current Opinion in Pharmacology* 17: 87–100. https://doi.org/10.1016/j.coph.2014.07.007.

Bushnell, D.L., M.T. Madsen, T. O'cdorisio, Y. Menda, S. Muzahir, R. Ryan, and M.S. O'dorisio. 2014. Feasibility and advantage of adding (131)I-MIBG to (90)Y-DOTATOC for treatment of patients with advanced stage neuroendocrine tumors. *EJNMMI Research* 4 (1): 38. https://doi.org/10.1186/s13550-014-0038-2. Epub 2014 Sep 10. PMID:26116109.

Cascante, M., et al. 2002. Metabolic control analysis in drug discovery and disease. *Nature Biotechnology* 20: 243–249. https://doi.org/10.1038/nbt0302-243.

Csermely, P. 2004. Strong links are important, but weak links stabilize them. *Trends in Biochemical Sciences* 29: 331–334. https://doi.org/10.1016/j.tibs.2004.05.004.

Csermely, P., V. Agoston, and S. Pongor. 2005. The efficiency of multi-target drugs: The network approach might help drug design. *Trends in Pharmacological Sciences* 26: 178–182. https://doi.org/10.1016/j.tips.2005.02.007.

Haberkorn, U., M. Eder, K. Kopka, J.W. Babich, and M. Eisenhut. 2016. New strategies in prostate cancer: Prostate-specific membrane antigen (PSMA) ligands for diagnosis and therapy. *Clinical Cancer Research* 22: 9–15. https://doi.org/10.1158/1078-0432.CCR-15-0820.

Haberkorn, U., W. Mier, K. Kopka, C. Herold-Mende, A. Altmann, and J. Babich. 2017. Identification of ligands and translation to clinical applications. *Journal of Nuclear Medicine* 58 (Suppl 2): 27S–33S. https://doi.org/10.2967/jnumed.116.186791.

Hassanzadeh, S., et al. 2010. Decision making under uncertainty in drug development. In *24th World Congress International Project Management Association*, 1. Istanbul: International Project Management Association. hal-00745303.

Head, G.L. 1967. An alternative to defining risk as uncertainty. *The Journal of Risk and Insurance* 34: 205–214. https://doi.org/10.2307/251319.

Iyengar, S.S., and M.R. Lepper. 2000. When choice is demotivating: Can one desire too much a good thing? *Journal of Personality and Social Psychology* 79: 995–1006. https://doi.org/10.1037/0022-3514.79.6.995.

Knight, F. 1921. *Risk, uncertainty and profit*. Ghe Riverside Press: Boston/New York. https://doi.org/10.1097/00000658-192112000-00004.

Korcsmaros, T., et al. 2007. How to design multi-target drugs: Target search options in cellular networks. *Expert Opinion on Drug Discovery* 2: 799–808. https://doi.org/10.1517/17460441.2.6.799.

Leibniz, G.W. 1704. *Nouveaux essais sur l'entendement humain*. Paris: Flammarion.

Levitin, F., O. Stern, M. Weiss, C. Gil-Henn, R. Ziv, Z. Prokocimer, N.I. Smorodinsky, D.B. Rubinstein, and D.H. Wreschner. 2005. The MUC1 SEA module is a self-cleaving domain. *The Journal of Biological Chemistry* 280: 33374–33386. https://doi.org/10.1074/jbc.M506047200.

Lindsay, M.A. 2003. Target discovery. *Nature Reviews Drug Discovery* 2: 831–838. https://doi.org/10.1038/nrd1202.

Lipton, S.A. 2004. Turning down, but not off. Neuroprotection requires a paradigm shift in drug development. *Nature* 428: 473. https://doi.org/10.1038/428473a.

Lhuillier, C., N.P. Rudqvist, O. Elemento, S.C. Formenti, and S. Demaria. 2019. Radiation therapy and anti-tumor immunity: Exposing immunogenic mutations to the immune system. *Genome Medicine* 11 (1): 40. https://doi.org/10.1186/s13073-019-0653-7.

Modos, D., et al. 2017. Neighbors of cancer-related proteins have key influence on pathogenesis and could increase the drug target space for anticancer therapies. *Systems Biology and Applications* 3: 2. https://doi.org/10.1038/s41540-017-0003-6.

Poste, G. 2011. Bring on the biomarkers. *Nature* 469: 156–157. https://doi.org/10.1038/469156a.

Pradet-Balade, B., F. Boulmé, H. Beug, E.W. Müllner, and J.A. Garcia-Sanz. 2001. Translation control: Bridging the gap between genomics and proteomics? *Trends in Biochemical Sciences* 26: 225–229. https://doi.org/10.1016/S0968-0004(00)01776-X.

Prinz, F., T. Schlange, and K. Asadullah. 2011. Believe it or not: How much can we rely on published data on potential drug targets? *Nature Reviews Drug Discovery* 10: 712. https://doi.org/10.1038/nrd3439-c1.

Rescher, N. 1960. Choice without preference. A study of the history and of the logic of Buridans ass. *Kant-Studien* 51: 142–175. https://doi.org/10.1515/kant.1960.51.1-4.142.

Rogawski, M.A. 2000. Low affinity channel blocking (uncompetitive) NMDA receptor antagonists as therapeutic agents – Towards an understanding of their favorable tolerability. *Amino Acids* 19: 133–149. https://doi.org/10.1007/s007260070042.

Rubinstein, D.B., M. Karmely, R. Ziv, I. Benhar, O. Leitner, S. Baron, B.Z. Katz, and D.H. Wreschner. 2006. MUC1/X protein immunization enhances cDNA immunization in generating anti-MUC1/junction antibodies that target malignant cells. *Cancer Research* 66: 11247–11253. https://doi.org/10.1158/0008-5472.CAN-06-1486.

Shenhav, A., and R.L. Buckner. 2014. Neural correlates of dueling affective reactions to win–win choices. *PNAS* 111: 10978–10983.

Sotiriou, C., and L. Pusztai. 2009. Gene-expression signatures in breast cancer. *The New England Journal of Medicine* 360: 790–800. https://doi.org/10.1056/NEJMra0801289.

Stock, J.K., N.P. Jones, T. Hammonds, J. Roffey, and C. Dillon. 2015. Adressing the right targets in oncology: Challenges and alternative approaches. *Journal of Biomolecular Screening* 20: 305–317. https://doi.org/10.1177/1087057114564349.

Stuart, J.M., et al. 2003. A gene-coexpression network for global discovery of conserved genetic modules. *Science* 302: 249–255. https://doi.org/10.1126/science.1087447.

Wall, T.D., J.L. Cordery, and C.W. Clegg. 2002. Empowerment, performance and operational uncertainty: A theoretical integration. *Applied Psychology* 51: 146–169. https://doi.org/10.1111/1464-0597.00083.

Watts, D.J., and S.H. Strogatz. 1998. Collective dynamics of 'small-world' networks. *Nature* 393: 440–442. https://doi.org/10.1038/30918.

Yap, T.A., M. Gerlinger, P.A. Futreal, L. Pusztai, and C. Swanton. 2012. Intratumoral heterogeneity: Seeing the wood for the trees. *Science Translational Medicine* 4: 1–4.

Wong, C.H., K.W. Siah, and A.W. Lo. 2018. Estimation of clinical trial success rates and related parameters. *Biostatistics* 14: 14–19.

Chapter 7
Medical Imaging and Artificial Intelligence

Luca Casini and Marco Roccetti

Abstract As with most aspects of our lives in the last few years, medicine too has seen the rise of Artificial Intelligence (AI) applications with an equal amount of fear and fascination from the mainstream public. Scientists, though, tend to be more cautious in their opinions towards these new technologies, as AI in its essence is not new at all and has already gained and lost popularity several times in the past. However, it is undeniable how Deep Learning (DL) has obtained incredible results that surpassed previously established standard procedures and has the potential to yield even better results. Still, this potential comes with some caveats that need to be pointed out to whoever wants to adopt this new paradigm. This chapter focuses on DL application in the world of medical imaging, providing basic notions in order to discuss the state of the art as well as bringing up some interesting issues and critical questions concerning medical application of AI.

Keywords Artificial intelligence · Deep learning · Medical imaging

7.1 Introduction

The aim of this chapter is to give a basic idea of AI and Deep Learning and to introduce examples of state-of-the-art applications in the field of medical imaging, as well as presenting some issues that the use of AI brings up.

In order to properly discuss the subject, we start by briefly retracing the history of AI, as the term has come to mean so many different things, and by defining some terminology and basic concepts of machine learning about data and training; then we will describe some more aspects specific to deep learning. This introductory section ends with a description of the staple neural network architectures for imaging tasks.

L. Casini (✉) · M. Roccetti
Department of Computer Science and Engineering, University of Bologna, Bologna, Italy
e-mail: luca.casini7@unibo.it; marco.roccetti@unibo.it

© The Author(s), under exclusive license to Springer Nature
Switzerland AG 2020
E. Lalumera, S. Fanti (eds.), *Philosophy of Advanced Medical Imaging*,
SpringerBriefs in Ethics, https://doi.org/10.1007/978-3-030-61412-6_7

81

In the second section, we will quickly discuss modern machine-based methods applied to various problems in the vast field of medical imaging, from detection and segmentation to image registration.

The third section is dedicated to the role of data and wants to highlight the importance of datasets for deep learning (and machine learning in general), and how any kind of bias and noise in the data can lead to serious problems if not addressed in the correct way.

Finally, the fourth section contains some reflections on the use of deep learning in medicine, its strengths and shortcomings (beyond what sensational headlines may lead to think) and what its integration in the health system may entail for physicians and patients.

7.1.1 Artificial Intelligence Is (Not) a Big Deal

In the last few years, Artificial Intelligence has become one of the hottest and most controversial topics of discussion, with opinions ranging from the enthusiastic and hopeful to the grim and dystopic. Many speak of a revolution that will completely change our lives forever (some would argue that it already did) but it is often the case that scientists are considerably more cautious with their expectations on these new technologies.

Part of the reason behind this is that AI is not as new as it seems; it may surprise the uninformed reader but the field is very old and dates back to the 1950s. Throughout the last 60 years it was characterized by various approaches and went in and out of fashion multiple times.

Early works were interested in making machines learn from data, thus the field named Machine Learning, using statistical and probabilistic methods and models. Some researchers also tried to create biologically inspired computational units, the precursors to the artificial neurons and neural networks that we use today, but soon encountered difficulties connected to the lack of computational power and also of algorithmic nature. In the 1970s, the enthusiasm decreased, and funding was pulled from many projects leading to the so called "AI winter".

In the 1980s, AI became synonymous with rule-based formal systems that were capable of inference starting from a structured knowledge base. Those systems, called expert systems, were quite capable and obtained commercial success, but required humans to precisely define the nature of the task and codify all the information.

Rule-based systems eventually went out of favor and in the 90s Machine Learning was making a comeback, pushed by the availability of computational power and advances on the algorithmic side. In the 2000s, with the increasing amount of data available, mostly thanks to the Internet, artificial neural networks finally had a chance to show their true potential and started becoming a standard in many problems; eventually a new discipline emerged called Deep Learning, that focused on the creation of neural network models that stacked many layers of neurons (hence the name) to solve machine learning problems.

Deep Learning has proved its usefulness and continues pushing the state of the art and enabling new technologies that were unthinkable before (Casini et al. 2018). The importance of this new discipline for computer science, and as a precious tool for any other field, is confirmed by the decision of the ACM (Association for Computing Machinery) to award the Turing Prize of 2018 to J. Bengio, G. Hinton and Y. LeCun, three of the most important scientists in the field that are considered the fathers of Deep Learning.

Still, given the history of artificial intelligence since its infancy, in the scientific community people tend not to get carried away by enthusiasm, even recognizing the impact of DL, as they understand that there are huge leaps forward to be made before we can think of true intelligent systems.

7.1.2 Basic Concepts and Terminology

The fundamental goal of **Machine Learning** (ML) is to create a machine able to carry out a task with increasing performance as it accumulates experience. In layman terms, this means we want to build a model that learns to do something directly from data, and the more it sees the better it gets.

The first part of a machine learning pipeline is gathering data and cleaning it by removing outliers and malformed data and transforming it into a format that is fit for the algorithm of choice. Once the dataset is ready, the Training phase can start. Training consists of showing the model examples and evaluating the output to measure its performance. This is done using a function that represents the goal of our task, called **Loss Function**, usually measuring how "off" the predictions are from the ground truth. This means that ML is basically just an optimization problem where we are adjusting our model parameters in an effort to minimize the loss function. Machine learning models are commonly trained in a batch fashion, presenting a subset of the training data at a time, and then correcting the model; this is needed because the dataset is usually bigger than the available working memory. A complete iteration over the training data is called an **Epoch**.

In order to estimate if the training is being carried out successfully a small part of the dataset (usually one tenth) is kept apart during training and used to verify the output, in a process called **Validation**. Once we are happy with our training, or more frequently when the loss function starts to plateau (which means performance is not increasing anymore), we can stop and move on to **Testing**; during this last phase we use data that the model has never seen before and evaluate its performance. This is a good estimate of what to expect in a real-world scenario (assuming that the test set was sampled correctly from the data). The necessity of using different data for evaluation stems from the fact that during training our model could have learned "by heart" how to treat each example, in what's called **Overfitting**, resulting in very high scores that do not translate to good performance once the machine is employed in the real world. The opposite situation, not having learned enough, is called **Underfitting**.

An important distinction we have to make is about the nature of the training process. Specifically, there are two major approaches called **Supervised** and

Unsupervised Learning. As the name suggests, Supervised methods entail some kind of human intervention, commonly in the form of labeled examples for the machine to look at. This category of models is usually faster to train and achieve better performance on specific tasks, but the downside is the added work necessary to gather labeled data and the lack of generality of the resulting model. Unsupervised methods, on the other hand, do not need labeled examples and learn how to make sense of the input data by looking at the data itself. Those methods can be useful to discover hidden relationships in the data that go unnoticed by human experts and in theory can create a model with a much more general representation of the world; but to do so they need a great quantity of data that may simply not be available.

Usually machine learning problems can be traced back to two types of fundamental tasks: **Classification** and **Regression**. Classification is the task of predicting to which class the input belongs to, learning how the data is divided, effectively finding the boundaries that separate each class. Regression, on the other hand, is the task of predicting some value given the inputs and, while classification can be argued to be specific case of regression, usually is used to refer to problems where it is necessary to predict the next value in a series or a continuous value like the price of something.

7.1.3   Deep Neural Networks and State of the Art Architectures

As anticipated in the Introduction, **Artificial Neural Networks** are not a novelty in the field of machine learning; what makes the difference this time is the word "deep", that we often hear along with "neural networks" and "learning", coming from the fact that modern neural networks are built by stacking many layers of neurons, thus becoming incredibly good at modeling complex relations hidden in big data.

Let us start by defining the artificial neuron, the basic unit of a neural network. Essentially, each neuron takes a vector of data as input and operates a weighted sum on it to obtain the output. This output is then fed to an **Activation Function** that simulates the "firing" of the neuron. While a single neuron is technically already a model able to make predictions, its modeling power is considerably limited, but many neurons side-by-side are already able to approximate any function. Stacking many rows of neurons, called layers, results in what is known as a **Deep Neural Network**.

The output of the neural network is compared with the expected output during the training phase in order to evaluate the error. This comparison is done using a function called Loss Function, with the objective of minimizing it. This optimization problem is tackled using gradient descent algorithms and, in turn, the network is adjusted to perform better in the process called **Backpropagation**. Effectively, what is being learned are the weights of the connections between neurons that are recomputed with every example that is shown to the network.

The most basic example of deep neural network is called **Multilayer Perceptron** (MLP), which is basically a network with at least three strongly connected layers (input, hidden and output layers), linked in a feed-forward fashion. These networks can approximate any function and are capable of decent performance in many tasks, but in the context of image analysis they show their limits as having a neuron for each pixel in the input quickly makes the number of parameters unmanageable.

Inspired by the functioning of the visual cortex, **Convolutional Neural Networks** (CNNs) were developed to overcome the limits of traditional neural networks in the context of image-based tasks (LeCun et al. 1989).

As in the brain, individual neurons fire to specific visual stimuli, so CNNs learn to recognize specific patterns wherever they appear. This "space invariance" is enabled by the convolution operation: a small matrix, called filter or kernel, is slid across the image (that is represented as a big matrix with a value corresponding to each pixel) and the dot product is computed. In CNNs the weights that are learned correspond to values in the filter and in each layer many different filters are learned, corresponding to specific feature extractors. The important part is that those weights are shared for each slice of the input during the sliding, greatly reducing the number of parameters to learn (this is known as parameter sharing) thus allowing space-invariance. CNNs can be tuned with respect to the dimensions and number of the filters, as well as to the stride of the sliding window (how many pixels are skipped in each step). After a convolutional layer, usually, there is a **Max-Pooling Layer**, which slides a window over its input and takes the max operation, resulting in a smaller feature map as the output. Pooling operations have the effect of increasing the so-called **Receptive Field**, effectively making the network learn higher level features as it gets deeper.

Some tasks involve looking at phenomena that happen over a period of time. To capture the information that is contained in the sequence of data points, and thus to learn the "temporal" relationship in the data, a special kind of neural networks is often used, called **Recurrent Neural Networks (RNNs)**. The idea behind this kind of network is that at each "timestep" the network is input with current data along with the output of the previous timestep. The most common implementation of RNNs are **Long Short-Term Memory (LSTM)** networks; they include a set of gated neurons that manage the network "memory" in order to avoid forgetting important things, as timesteps go by and the contribution of each becomes smaller and smaller.

7.2 Deep Learning for Medical Imaging

Interesting now is to discuss how deep neural networks can be leveraged in the field of medical imaging, with special attention to the subsequent tasks of classification, localization, segmentation, reconstruction, and computer-aided diagnosis.

7.2.1 Classification

Classification tasks are the most common problems in image processing with neural networks, even outside the field of medicine, and have been extensively researched. They consist in separating a set of images over to different groups based on a specific property that each image can either possess or not. This can either mean separating positive and negative exams or identify what type of tissue/lesion/organ is in the image. Medical imaging, however, poses some interesting challenges that may not emerge in other contexts. The main issue is the scarcity of labeled data to work with. While data augmentation can be useful in mitigating the issue, a more consistent solution is found in a novel technique called **Transfer Learning**. It consists of taking a model trained on a different, but similar, kind of data and fine-tune it for the new problem at hand. Esteva et al. (2017) have used a sophisticated CNN created by Google, called Inception v3 (Szegedy et al. 2016), and fine-tuned it to recognize skin cancer with performances close to those of human medics; more recent studies with a similar architecture, like ResNets (He et al. 2016), even managed to outperform specialists (Brinker et al. 2019; Hekler et al. 2019; Haenssle et al. 2018).

7.2.2 Localization

Sometimes there is a need to pinpoint where specific organs or landmarks are located in the image space (and time) as a step in the diagnostic process, or to support other techniques like segmentation. The problem is usually formulated as a classification problem: a pixel (or voxel in 3D) is either part of the landmark or not, resulting in a bounding box, or a mask, for the region of interest. Since working in 3D is not as easy as pie, most methods choose to extrapolate the location from a composition of 2D slices (D. Yang et al. 2015; de Vos et al. 2016). Using a different approach, localization can also be modeled as a regression problem, where the objective is predicting directly the coordinates of the landmark (Payer et al. 2016). Often the localization task involves temporal data in the form of consecutive images, or a video; in order to retain this temporal information, RNNs can be put to good use in conjunction with CNNs (Kong et al. 2016): the latter extracts features from the images and the former puts them in relation across time.

7.2.3 Segmentation

Segmentation is the task of outlining and separating important parts in an image and is a very critical issues for many fields that have a visual component, for example it represents one of the key challenges for individuating objects in the context of autonomous driving. In the field of medical imaging, it is an important step that enables further analysis by extracting data about volume, shape, number (think of cells), etc. from several sources, subjected to high variation. The state of the art of segmentation architectures is represented by U-Net (Ronneberger et al. 2015). The particularity of the model is that it employs inverse convolutions to scale back up the image after all the pooling layers, in order to recreate an image of the same size as the input, with every object comprising the original image highlighted as a separate item. The name comes from the fact that there is a downsampling branch going down, a bottleneck in the middle and, finally, an upsampling branch going up in the shape of an U. The final touch are the connections that go across the network, from each level of a branch to the corresponding one on the other branch, in order to retain the information lost in the downsampling. The original U-net was used for cell segmentation, but the architecture was used in other contexts like, for example, 3D MRI scans of prostate (Milletari et al. 2016) and kidneys (Çiçek et al. 2016).

7.2.4 Registration

Often overlooked, image registration is the process of taking images from multiple sources that represent the same subject and align them, allowing to gather information from all the different kinds of inputs, and to combine them effectively. It can also indicate data of the same subject from a single source that is collected overtime; in this case the registration process allows the physician to evaluate the evolution of a phenomenon. While other tasks based on visual recognition have benefited more from the introduction of DL, registration has not received as much attention, even though new research looks promising and offers comparable results with reduced computational load. Registration is usually approached with unsupervised learning models, like autoencoders. A common approach is to use deep learning to extract representative points for alignment and then use a classic method to align those points. Wu et al. (2013), for example, used convolutional autoencoders to extract better features and fed them to known algorithms (Demons, HAMMER), thus improving state-of-the-art performance in 3D image registration. Also, X. Yang et al. (2017b) designed an end-to-end model that effectively learns to approximate exact analytical methods, achieving registration with greater speed at the cost of a small error.

7.2.5 Reconstruction, Enhancement and Generation

AI can also be used to reconstruct or enhance the quality of an image. An example is combining multiple inputs of scarce quality to get a better image, removing noise, increasing the resolution of images (super resolution), etc. It is even possible to create new images altogether. Reconstruction can be achieved with traditional methods, but it is quite time consuming. AI can reduce the computational load by resorting to unsupervised methods that just learn how to minimize reconstruction errors. For example, Schlemper et al. (2018) used CNNs for reconstructing MR images with a great increase in speed. W. Yang et al. (2017a) used CNNs to hide bones in chest radiographs. Nie et al. (2017) used Generative Adversarial Networks (GAN) (a particular neural architecture where two network fight each other, one generates images and one tries to guess if they are fake) to create CT scans from MRIs, avoiding the patient radiation exposure. Similarly, Q. Yang et al. (2018) used GANs to reduce noise in low-dose CT images. Finally, Oktay et al. (2016) proposed a model that takes in2D chest scans and creates 3D images with super resolution. As Huang et al. (2018) showed, however, image reconstruction methods can lack the robustness needed; for example, noisy input can lead to deformation in the output, added artifacts, and even missing area of interest (like lesions). Precision Learning, the idea of integrating traditional analytical models in the neural architecture can be a solution every time a deterministic model can be either more effective, or less costly, than letting a machine learning through a stochastic process (Würfl et al. 2018).

7.2.6   Computer-Aided Diagnosis

Full automation of the diagnostic process is an interesting perspective and many medical applications of AI seem to point towards this utopian goal. Technology, however, is not yet there and chances are that it may never be. More convincing efforts are instead focused on supporting physicians along the process of diagnosis. This seems to be a more profitable way to go as AI can lighten the physician work-load by taking care of easy and automatable tasks in the decision process, so that humans can focus their attention to more challenging exams and cases. For example, an approach that can be used in any context where classification is performed is to consider the probabilistic output of the neural network and define a certain threshold for high confidence predictions of positive and negative cases. The remaining items that are classified with a probability below the threshold are left as dubious for the human expert to look at. This technique can be tuned to expect a specific number of errors (false positive and false negatives) in exchange for a bigger "gray zone" that humans will have to manage; still, having a reduced workload is always helpful, however small the reduction (Roccetti et al. 2019a). There are a number of examples of ML-supported Diagnosis in literature, directed to various specialists, like derma-tologists (Esteva et al. 2017), ophthalmologists (De Fauw et al. 2018) and radiolo-gists (Diamant et al. 2017). A common theme that emerges is that, while ML can help increase the diagnostic performance of medical doctors (especially for routine exams that require a lot of work), there is a need for explainable systems that can highlight evidence towards a decision. In addition, medical specialist must be aware of the limits of the conceptual limits of AI, as the "interpretation" of the machine is bound by the interpretation offered in the dataset and any lack of consensus on this is carried over. (Lalumera et al. 2019).

7.3 Dataset Issues

In the world of machine learning is clear how the role of data is of the utmost importance, nonetheless, is not rare to see models fail due to lack of care in the creation and manipulation of the dataset used during training. In a context like medical images, where different fields and specializations intersect, it is important that those who use DL tools with big data are conscious about the probabilistic nature of the mechanism, thus providing a correct interpretation to the results they obtain, not disregarding any bias that similar models can carry over.

7.3.1 Datasets: Quality vs. Quantity

The first issue to be addressed here is the, seemingly paradoxical, phenomenon where **more data does not equal better performance**. This is quite common in scenarios where whoever takes decisions wants to leverage the power of big data, driven by it being the buzzword of the moment, without realizing that not all data holds the same value. In particular, it is fundamental that a dataset is as clean from noise as much possible. These cleaning operations cannot be done without the intervention of the specialists (in this case physicians) that are the ones who know the domain. Disregarding this factor may lead to unpredictable outcomes (Casini et al. 2019; Roccetti et al. 2019b).

7.3.2 Imbalanced Dataset

One of the biggest issues in medicine is given by the case of Dataset Imbalance. In layman terms, certain phenomena, like diseases, are quite uncommon, relative to the dimension of the population, and one could argue that the more a phenomenon is interesting the rarer it is. There are techniques to combat this problem that consists in creating more data for the minority classes (Data augmentation and oversampling) or in reducing the difference, by discarding some data for the most numerous classes (undersampling). **Oversampling** and **Undersampling** can be operated in combination to mitigate the negative effects of both but they still modify the nature of the data that is being learned, thus introducing errors, albeit quantifiable, that researchers would gladly avoid. **Data augmentation**, on the other hand, is the process of creating new realistic examples starting from the existing data in a way that is not as artificial. A classic example is to mirror and rotate the images in a dataset as convolutional neural networks will treat those cases as something different. This operation does not affect the dataset properties in a meaningful way yet reinforces its learning potential.

7.3.3 Biased Datasets

Lastly, it is worth mentioning how in the process of building or analyzing a dataset is important to look out for any kind of bias. If a bias is evident in the dataset, but is not possible to obtain any more data, then it is important to recognize the limits of that model in order to avoid, potentially dangerous, errors. There are examples of racially biased systems in the law enforcement (Rudin 2019), voice and facial recognition. While a phone that does not unlock for dark skinned people is embarrassing but does not threaten the life of anyone, a system that gives harsher sentences to minorities or that gives wrong medical advice, because it was trained only on white people, represents serious danger for society. Thus, great care is required when designing systems of this kind. There have already been critical situations of gender biases (Risberg et al. 2009) as well as racial biases (Hall et al. 2015) in medical applications. If the start is not good, the machine will follow even deteriorating the situation (Cabitza et al. 2019). This means that those biases must not easily slip into the process of data gathering for training a machine, as this will result, in turn, in machine-based biased predictions. A biased machine model is a severe hazard as it may influence medical doctors in their human decision, in a vicious circle.

7.4 Beyond Technical Aspects

In the previous section we showed some criticalities that specifically concern data and that can hinder the progress and adoption of AI-based techniques in the field of medicine. However, there are also some problems that go beyond the technicalities of machine learning and that need to be addressed before AI-based solution can be automated something so delicate as healthcare.

Humans make mistakes and so do doctors. Medical errors and misdiagnosis area serious problem that silently takes its toll on patients (Makary and Daniel 2016; Neale et al. 2011) but AI could help resolve or, at the very least, mitigate. Considering this, a future of automated diagnosis and intervention would be something to look forward too. Unfortunately for automation enthusiasts, the human factor is something that will hardly be removed from the equation of healthcare. Part of the job of a doctor is to be able to understand this human factor that is at the basis of the relationship with the patient. A machine would not be able to communicate in such a way with a human and, in the case of a mistake, would be judged way harshly because of the lack of empathy. A similar reaction can be seen with how the public is perceiving driverless cars. It is not uncommon to hear people that are against them because they want to be in control and, even if they understand that there would likely be less accidents, they irrationally prefer to risk more and have humans driving. This makes sense both on the plane of trust and empathy, but also when considering the issue of responsibility; in the event of an accident knowing who to blame is reassuring, and AI cannot provide this.

The issue of **responsibility** may be the biggest problem with the applicability of DL-based solutions, not only in medicine, and relates to another problem, **explainability**. Deep learning is often described as a black box, a system that cannot be understood in its inner workings but just evaluated for its inputs and outputs. This means that when the output of the model is wrong, or leads to an incorrect decision, there is no way of finding out why exactly that mistake was made. If something goes wrong, whose fault is it? The physician that used the software or the company that designed it? Maybe neither, as everything was done correctly, and the case fell in the low percentage of error? The only way to answer a question like this is to have a model designed to be explainable from the start, as attempting to do it afterwards can introduce even more errors (Rudin 2019). The impossibility of explaining decision is the reason why AI-systems are marketed and utilized only as decision support in order to avoid any legal liability when things go wrong.

The current paradigm thus is centered around collaboration. This may be due to the impossibility of completely automating but perhaps it could be the better road to take. Collaboration is considered by many experts the best way of integrating AI in medicine (Miller and Brown 2018; Sim 2016) as it enables physicians to do their work better without sacrificing the best qualities of a human. As Chang (Chang 2019) noted, the work of a doctor is comprised of cognition and perception tasks. While AI excels at perception and is surpassing humans, on the cognition side there is a lot that leaves to be desired in terms of creative problem solving and decision-making. When considering the scenario of physicians using AI as a tool that helps them do a better job, we must not ignore that physicians can play an active role in improving the performance of the system too. Among the most promising methods to foster a cooperation between human specialists and learning machines is gaining prominence the one called Interactive Machine Learning (Holzinger 2016). The idea is having a human in the learning loop that, besides being the user, can also help the model improve, for example by selecting the most relevant and challenging images from the dataset to focus the learning effort.

This collaboration must be built on top of an exchange of knowledge between AI researchers and medical doctors. Who design systems for healthcare must know as much as possible of the process in order to avoid mistakes like the ones we talked previously but it is equally important for physicians to know how to treat the output of AI-based models so that they can get the most out of them. About this, there is evidence of automation bias in medical doctors when it comes to computer aided diagnosis. Bond et al. (Bond et al. 2018) experimented with ECG interpretation and showed that when doctors correct interpretation differed from the wrong output of the AI, they tended to follow the machine advice and this undermined their confidence and thus their performance (non-cardiologists were more affected than cardiologists).

In conclusion, while is interesting and important to think about a future of automated healthcare in general we find that envisioning and working towards a world of collaboration between human specialists and AI-based models is much more profitable and can lead to great results in the next few years.

7.5   Conclusion

Deep Learning is undoubtedly one of the greatest breakthroughs in technology and science in the last decade and new Artificial Intelligence systems powered by it are going to be more and more present in our lives. We tried to give some perspective on a field that is older than most people would think by quickly telling its history followed by a brief overview of how the inner workings of those systems, where we pointed out some of the strengths and weaknesses of DL models. Knowing how the field came to be is important to avoid the influence of overly enthusiastic promises made by some researchers and the hype that is fostered by some press in the tech world. Knowing how deep learning is working under the hood is very useful for those who will use it as a tool because it can help finding problems and avoiding pitfalls.

We then gave a few significant examples of state-of-the-art applications in the context of medical imaging to show how DL and AI are now the weapon of choice for a vast number of use cases in the field. It is clear that, aside from philosophical considerations, the hindrance to the progress of machine learning in the world of medicine is the availability of data and its quality. We find that it is never stressed enough how important data gathering and preparation is to the performance of artificial intelligence systems. Datasets are both the fuel of the deep learning engine and, in a sense, the steering wheel because they condition the performance of a model but also encode the question the model is trying to answer. Badly structured data and targets may result in a good model that performs badly because it is actually fit for the wrong task.

Finally, we took some time to express a few thoughts on some critical aspects of this field that go beyond the technical part. Artificial intelligence and big data open up a Pandoras box of potential issues from privacy to the actual responsibility of AI decision. Given our experience, we wanted to point in the direction of a collaboration between AI and human professionals that can leverage the best characteristics of both: the capacity of harnessing unmanageable amounts of data to gather new insights of AI and the flexibility and specificity of the human intellect.

References

Bond, Raymond R., Tomas Novotny, Irena Andrsova, Lumir Koc, Martina Sisakova, Dewar Finlay, Daniel Guldenring, et al. 2018. Automation Bias in medicine: The influence of automated diagnoses on interpreter accuracy and uncertainty when Reading electrocardiograms. *Journal of Electrocardiology* 51 (6): S6–S11.

Brinker, Titus J., Achim Hekler, Alexander H. Enk, Joachim Klode, Axel Hauschild, Carola Berking, Bastian Schilling, et al. 2019. Deep learning outperformed 136 of 157 dermatologists in a head-to-head Dermoscopic melanoma image classification task. *European Journal of Cancer* 113: 47–54.

Cabitza, Federico, Andrea Campagner, and Davide Ciucci. 2019. New frontiers in explainable AI: understanding the GI to interpret the GO. In *International cross-domain conference for machine learning and knowledge extraction*, 27–47. Berlin Heidelberg: Springer.

Casini, Luca, Gustavo Marfia, and Marco Roccetti. 2018. Some reflections on the potential and limitations of deep learning for automated music generation. In *2018 IEEE 29th annual international symposium on personal, indoor and mobile radio communications (PIMRC)*, 27–31. Bologna: PIMRC. https://doi.org/10.1109/PIMRC.2018.8581038.

Casini, Luca, Giovanni Delnevo, Marco Roccetti, Nicolò Zagni, and Giuseppe Cappiello. 2019. Deep water: predicting water meter failures through a human-machine intelligence collaboration. In *International conference on human interaction and emerging technologies*, 688–694. Berlin Heidelberg: Springer.

Chang, Anthony. 2019. Common misconceptions and future directions for AI in medicine: A physician-data scientist perspective. In *Conference on Artificial Intelligence in Medicine in Europe, 3–6*. Pavia: Springer.

Çiçek, Özgün, Ahmed Abdulkadir, Soeren S. Lienkamp, Thomas Brox, and Olaf Ronneberger. 2016. 3D U-Net: Learning dense volumetric segmentation from sparse annotation. In *International Conference on Medical Image Computing and Computer-Assisted Intervention*, 424–432. Cambridge: Springer.

De Fauw, Jeffrey, Joseph R. Ledsam, Bernardino Romera-Paredes, Stanislav Nikolov, Nenad Tomasev, Sam Blackwell, Harry Askham, et al. 2018. Clinically applicable deep learning for diagnosis and referral in retinal disease. *Nature Medicine* 24 (9): 1342.

de Vos, Bob D., Jelmer M. Wolterink, Pim A. de Jong, Max A. Viergever, and Ivana Išgum. 2016. 2D image classification for 3D anatomy localization: Employing deep convolutional neural networks. In *Medical Imaging 2016: Image Processing, 9784:97841Y*. Bellingham: International Society for Optics and Photonics.

Diamant, Idit, Yaniv Bar, Ofer Geva, Lior Wolf, Gali Zimmerman, Sivan Lieberman, Eli Konen, and Hayit Greenspan. 2017. Chest radiograph pathology categorization via transfer learning. In *Deep learning for medical image analysis*, 299–320. New York: Elsevier.

Esteva, Andre, Brett Kuprel, Roberto A. Novoa, Justin Ko, Susan M. Swetter, Helen M. Blau, and Sebastian Thrun. 2017. Dermatologist-level classification of skin cancer with deep neural networks. *Nature* 542 (7639): 115–118. https://doi.org/10.1038/nature21056.

Haenssle, Holger A., Christine Fink, R. Schneiderbauer, Ferdinand Toberer, Timo Buhl, A. Blum, A. Kalloo, et al. 2018. Man against machine: Diagnostic performance of a deep learning convolutional neural network for dermoscopic melanoma recognition in comparison to 58 dermatologists. *Annals of Oncology* 29 (8): 1836–1842.

Hall, William J., Mimi V. Chapman, Kent M. Lee, Yesenia M. Merino, Tainayah W. Thomas, B. Keith Payne, Eugenia Eng, Steven H. Day, and Tamera Coyne-Beasley. 2015. Implicit racial/ethnic bias among health care professionals and its influence on health care outcomes: A systematic review. *American Journal of Public Health* 105 (12): e60–e76.

He, Kaiming, Xiangyu Zhang, Shaoqing Ren, and Jian Sun. 2016. Deep residual learning for image recognition. In *The IEEE Conference on Computer Vision and Pattern Recognition (CVPR)*. Ithaca: Cornell University.

Hekler, Achim, Jochen S. Utikal, Alexander H. Enk, Wiebke Solass, Max Schmitt, Joachim Klode, Dirk Schadendorf, et al. 2019. Deep learning outperformed 11 pathologists in the classification of histopathological melanoma images. *European Journal of Cancer* 118: 91–96.

Holzinger, Andreas. 2016. Interactive machine learning for health informatics: When do we need the human-in-the-loop? *Brain Informatics* 3 (2): 119–131.

Huang, Yixing, Tobias Würfl, Katharina Breininger, Ling Liu, Günter Lauritsch, and Andreas Maier. 2018. Some investigations on robustness of deep learning in limited angle tomography. In *International Conference on Medical Image Computing and Computer-Assisted Intervention*, 145–153. San Diego: Springer.

Kong, Bin, Yiqiang Zhan, Min Shin, Thomas Denny, and Shaoting Zhang. 2016. Recognizing end-diastole and end-systole frames via deep temporal regression network. In *International*

Conference on Medical Image Computing and Computer-Assisted Intervention, 264–272. Athens: Springer.

Lalumera, Elisabetta, Stefano Fanti, and Giovanni Boniolo. 2019. Reliability of molecular imaging diagnostics. *Synthese*. https://doi.org/10.1007/s11229-019-02419-y.

LeCun, Y., B. Boser, J.S. Denker, D. Henderson, R.E. Howard, W. Hubbard, and L.D. Jackel. 1989. Backpropagation applied to handwritten zip code recognition. *Neural Computation* 1 (4): 541–551. https://doi.org/10.1162/neco.1989.1.4.541.

Makary, Martin A., and Michael Daniel. 2016. Medical error—The third leading cause of death in the US. *BMJ* 353: i2139.

Miller, D. Douglas, and Eric W. Brown. 2018. Artificial intelligence in medical practice: The question to the answer? *The American Journal of Medicine* 131 (2): 129–133.

Milletari, Fausto, Nassir Navab, and Seyed-Ahmad Ahmadi. 2016. V-Net: Fully convolutional neural networks for volumetric medical image segmentation. In *2016 Fourth International Conference on 3D Vision (3DV)*, 565–571. Munich: IEEE.

Neale, Graham, Helen Hogan, and Nick Sevdalis. 2011. Misdiagnosis: Analysis based on case record review with proposals aimed to improve diagnostic processes. *Clinical Medicine* 11 (4): 317–321.

Nie, Dong, Roger Trullo, Jun Lian, Caroline Petitjean, Su Ruan, Qian Wang, and Dinggang Shen. 2017. Medical image synthesis with context-aware generative adversarial networks. In *International Conference on Medical Image Computing and Computer-Assisted Intervention*, 417–425. Lima: Springer.

Oktay, Ozan, Wenjia Bai, Matthew Lee, Ricardo Guerrero, Konstantinos Kamnitsas, Jose Caballero, Antonio de Marvao, Stuart Cook, Declan O'Regan, and Daniel Rueckert. 2016. Multi-input cardiac image super-resolution using convolutional neural networks. In *International Conference on Medical Image Computing and Computer-Assisted Intervention*, 246–254. Lima: Springer.

Payer, Christian, Darko Štern, Horst Bischof, and Martin Urschler. 2016. Regressing heatmaps for multiple landmark localization using CNNs. In *International Conference on Medical Image Computing and Computer-Assisted Intervention*, 230–238. Lima: Springer.

Risberg, Gunilla, Eva E. Johansson, and Katarina Hamberg. 2009. A theoretical model for analysing gender bias in medicine. *International Journal for Equity in Health* 8 (1): 28.

Roccetti, Marco, Giovanni Delnevo, Luca Casini, and Giuseppe Cappiello. 2019a. Is bigger always better? A controversial journey to the Center of Machine Learning Design, with uses and misuses of big data for predicting water meter failures. *Journal of Big Data* 6 (1): 70. https://doi.org/10.1186/s40537-019-0235-y.

Roccetti, Marco, Giovanni Delnevo, Luca Casini, Nicolò Zagni, and Giuseppe Cappiello. 2019b. A paradox in ML design: Less data for a smarter water metering cognification experience. In *Proceedings of the 5th EAI International Conference on Smart Objects and Technologies for Social Good*, GoodTechs '19, 201–206. Valencia: Association for Computing Machinery. https://doi.org/10.1145/3342428.3342685.

Ronneberger, Olaf, Philipp Fischer, and Thomas Brox. 2015. U-Net: Convolutional networks for biomedical image segmentation. In *International Conference on Medical Image Computing and Computer-Assisted Intervention*, 234–241. Peru: Springer.

Rudin, Cynthia. 2019. Stop explaining black box machine learning models for high stakes decisions and use interpretable models instead. *Nature Machine Intelligence* 1 (5): 206–215. https://doi.org/10.1038/s42256-019-0048-x.

Schlemper, Jo, Daniel C. Castro, Wenjia Bai, Chen Qin, Ozan Oktay, Jinming Duan, Anthony N. Price, Jo Hajnal, and Daniel Rueckert. 2018. Bayesian deep learning for accelerated MR image reconstruction. In *International Workshop on Machine Learning for Medical Image Reconstruction*, 64–71. Peru: Springer.

Sim, Ida. 2016. Two ways of knowing: Big data and evidence-based medicine. *Annals of Internal Medicine* 164 (8): 562–563.

Szegedy, Christian, Vincent Vanhoucke, Sergey Ioffe, Jon Shlens, and Zbigniew Wojna. 2016. Rethinking the inception architecture for computer vision. In *Proceedings of the IEEE Conference on Computer Vision and Pattern Recognition*, 2818–2826.

Wu, Guorong, Minjeong Kim, Qian Wang, Yaozong Gao, Shu Liao, and Dinggang Shen. 2013. Unsupervised deep feature learning for deformable registration of MR brain images. In *International Conference on Medical Image Computing and Computer-Assisted Intervention*, 649–656. Lima: Springer.

Würfl, Tobias, Mathis Hoffmann, Vincent Christlein, Katharina Breininger, Yixin Huang, Mathias Unberath, and Andreas K. Maier. 2018. Deep learning computed tomography: Learning projection-domain weights from image domain in limited angle problems. *IEEE Transactions on Medical Imaging* 37 (6): 1454–1463.

Yang, Dong, Shaoting Zhang, Zhennan Yan, Chaowei Tan, Kang Li, and Dimitris Metaxas. 2015. Automated anatomical landmark detection ondistal femur surface using convolutional neural network. In *2015 IEEE 12th International Symposium on Biomedical Imaging (ISBI)*, 17–21. Paris: IEEE.

Yang, Wei, Yingyin Chen, Yunbi Liu, Liming Zhong, Genggeng Qin, Zhentai Lu, Qianjin Feng, and Wufan Chen. 2017a. Cascade of multi-scale convolutional neural networks for bone suppression of chest radiographs in gradient domain. *Medical Image Analysis* 35: 421–433.

Yang, Xiao, Roland Kwitt, Martin Styner, and Marc Niethammer. 2017b. Quicksilver: Fast predictive image registration–a deep learning approach. *NeuroImage* 158: 378–396.

Yang, Qingsong, Pingkun Yan, Yanbo Zhang, Hengyong Yu, Yongyi Shi, Xuanqin Mou, Mannudeep K. Kalra, Yi Zhang, Ling Sun, and Ge Wang. 2018. Low-dose CT image denoising using a generative adversarial network with Wasserstein distance and perceptual loss. *IEEE Transactions on Medical Imaging* 37 (6): 1348–1357.

Part III
Ethics

Chapter 8
Overutilization of Imaging Tests and Healthcare Fairness

Kristin Bakke Lysdahl and Bjørn Hofmann

Abstract The aim of this chapter is to discuss the phenomenon of overutilization of imaging tests with respect to healthcare fairness. Before entering the discussion of fairness, we will briefly outline the concept of overutilization, and the scope and drivers of the phenomenon. We will end the chapter by indicating some potential solutions to combat overutilization of imaging tests.

Keywords Medical imaging · Overutilization · Fairness · Ethics

8.1 Introduction

Overutilization of radiological examination is not a new concern. In fact, it has been addressed in scientific literature for at least 4 decades (Hall 1976; Abrams 1979). One reason for this is the fascination for the technology that enable us to see pathologic processes directly (Kevles 1997). The radiologic aphorism of: "One look is worth a thousand listens" (Gunderman 2005), reduced the role of history taking, external signs and physical examination of the patient as diagnostic tools, in favour of imaging examinations. X-ray examinations were reported to be "regularly performed when an accurate diagnosis can be made with the naked eye, ear or finger" (McClenahan 1970). Throughout the latest decades, the development in medical imaging technologies is overwhelming. This technological progress reinforces the powerful belief that "the body can be simply seen through and the diseases

K. B. Lysdahl (✉)
Faculty of Health and Social Sciences, University of South-Eastern Norway, Drammen, Norway
e-mail: Kristin.Bakke.Lysdahl@usn.no

B. Hofmann
Norwegian University of Science and Technology, Gjøvik, Norway

Centre for Medical Ethics, University of Oslo, Oslo, Norway
e-mail: bjoern.hofmann@ntnu.no

E. Lalumera, S. Fanti (eds.), *Philosophy of Advanced Medical Imaging*, SpringerBriefs in Ethics, https://doi.org/10.1007/978-3-030-61412-6_8

recognized by the doctor's impartial gaze" (Lalumera et al. 2019). Unfortunately, this is a false belief, as imaging tests are neither immediate nor infallible, but the illusion that with a PET or a CT scan doctors directly see the disease may explain why overutilization is a persistent problem (ibid). The aim of this chapter is to discuss the phenomenon of overutilization of imaging tests with respect to healthcare fairness. Before entering the discussion of fairness, we will briefly outline the concept of overutilization, and the scope and drivers of the phenomenon. We will end the chapter by indicating some potential solutions to combat overutilization of imaging tests.

8.2 Defining Overutilization

Overutilization is but one of many concepts used to describe excessive or "too much" imaging (Hofmann 2010). While other concepts that address the issue of excess highlight various issues, such as usefulness ("non-productive"), need ("unnecessary"), safety ("overexposure"), morals ("inappropriate"), and lack of control ("indiscriminate use"), overutilization address both amount and utility (Otero et al. 2006). Lack of utility is a central feature of overutilization, which includes aspects of usefulness and need. In the medical context overutilization are understood as examinations not useful or not needed in the sense that they are deemed unlikely to contribute clinically to the patient's treatment (Blachar et al. 2006). A related term is *low-value care*, which refers to an "intervention in which evidence suggests it confers no or very little benefit for the patients, or risk of harm exceeds probable benefit, or more broadly, the added costs of the intervention do not provide proportional added benefits" (Elshaug et al. 2017). Terms like *inappropriate* or *not indicated* imaging are frequently used, reflecting that the main concern embedded in overutilization is the missing/marginal benefits or clinical value of the examination.

Overutilization is also increasingly being addressed in the radiation protection context, where it is related to the concept (and principle) of *justification*. The principle of justification states that application of a particular procedure to an individual patient should be judged to do more good than harm (Clement and Ogino 2018). In the radiation protection context overutilization is first and foremost a safety issue where harms in focus are the radiation detriment that the examinations may cause. However, the justification principle require consideration of benefits, costs and negative consequences to the individual patient as well as society (Clement and Ogino 2018). Hence, the radiation protection perspective also includes a utility issue, in terms of waste of healthcare costs and resources in society. Overutilization understood as an issue of waste and futility is a most relevant perspective when addressing the fairness below.

In this chapter we will limit the understanding of overutilization to entire tests/ examinations, requested and performed. It can be argued that too many projections and retakes can be classified as overutilization. However, to also address overutilization caused by how examinations are carried out is a question of optimization of procedures and beyond the scope here, as the question of justice mainly concerns providing and receiving imaging services or not.

Irrespective of what we emphasize in our understanding of overutilization it should be noticed that a single examination can be classified as overutilization only in retrospect, when the outcome is known. Besides, the outcome can be hard to determine because of the time spend as well as the various actions and incidents between the examination and the final health outcome. These facts of uncertainty make overutilization a highly complex phenomenon to define, determine, measure, and assess.

8.3 Mapping Overutilization

Investigating overutilization rates are by no means straightforward, reflecting the lack of clear distinctions between medically appropriate and inappropriate examinations. Still the number of empirical studies of unwarranted radiological examination are continuously growing, aiming to determining the extent of inappropriate radiological examination.

These studies use a variety of methods. A rough idea of the potential extension of overutilization based on referral quality can be obtained by asking radiographers and radiologists to state the proportion of examinations they approve out of those they are requested to justify (Koutalonis and Horrocks 2012). Most studies on the extension of overutilization are based on assessments of the referrals compliance with guidelines/imaging pathways. For instance a Finnish study found only 24% of the cervical, 46% of the thoracic, and 32% of the lumbar spine radiography referrals were in compliance with guidelines before the interventions (Tahvonen et al. 2017) and an Australian study found 40% of emergency department x-ray examination was deemed unnecessary not meeting an imaging pathway (Rawle and Pighills 2018). The underlying moral values in such approaches to measuring overutilization is conformity to professional norms and standards. Two other approaches investigate whether the examination solves the referrer's clinical problem (Simpson and Hartrick 2007) or whether the examination affects the subsequent management of the patients (Lehnert and Bree 2010). The moral value embedded in these approaches is normally the utility for the referring physicians or efficient health care, in terms of economic impact (Adams et al. 2018), i.e. a society perspective of usefulness and waste. However, few studies investigate the outcome of overutilization on patient health.

The investigation of overuse may also differ with respect to scope, focusing on a single modality or specific examination, for example: CT examinations (Almén et al. 2009) and spine radiography (Tahvonen et al. 2017). Moreover, the studies may only investigate referrals from limited practice settings, e.g. primary care or emergency department. These and other variations in research methods make it difficult to determine and accurately compare rates of overutilization of examinations across institutions and geographical areas. Keeping these scientific uncertainties in mind, overall overutilization is roughly estimated to be about ¼ of all radiological examination in developed countries.

8.4   Drivers of Overutilization

We started this chapter with mentioning one of the main drivers of overutilization of imaging, i.e. the fascination of the amazing technology and its apparent infallibility. This means that characteristics of the technology itself and how it is apprehended by us can lead to overutilization. The appeal of high-tech imaging can be explained by our intuitive beliefs, which tells us that "[m]ore is better, new is better, more expensive is better, and technology is good (Saini et al. 2017) or that "earlier is always better than late" (Hofmann and Skolbekken 2017). Hence we will opt for one examination too many rather than one too few.

These beliefs are examples of drivers of over- and underuse of health-care resources in general that also apply to overutilization of imaging. They belong to the first of three identified domains: (a) knowledge, bias, and uncertainty; (b) money and finance; and (c) power and human relationships (Saini et al. 2017). Just to give a few examples with domain (b) fee-for-service or volume-based payments encourage the provision, and poor coordination of services delivered to individual patient can lead to duplication of services. Regarding domain (c) imbalance of power and lack of trust in the patient-clinician relationship can cause overutilization as well as underuse (ibid). Figure 8.1 gives an overview of some of the drivers of overutilization.

We will not go into further details here. The main point is that drivers of overutilization make up a highly complex picture, as all domains operate at the global, national, regional, and individual level and a multiplicity of single factor are interacting. A number of stakeholders are ascribed responsibility: patients, next of kin, clinicians, administrators, payers and health policy makers. In imaging, radiologists and radiographers add up the number of stakeholders, and increases the complexity. We will return to a discussion of their role in the final section. The point here is that to address and reduce overutilization we need to identify its drivers and stakeholders.

8.5   Overutilization and Fairness

Overutilization of diagnostic imaging is intuitively incompatible with fairness. In order to better understand this intuition, we will in the following outline three theoretical perspectives of fairness: the egalitarian, the utilitarian, and the contractarian, and illuminate why overutilization is inconsistent with them all. According to Rawls fairness and justice are different (because fairness is the fundamental idea of the concept of justice). However, for the topic of this paper we do not need to distinguish between fairness and justice.

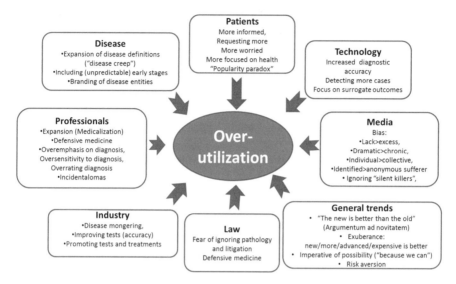

Fig. 8.1 Overview of some of the drivers of overutilization, based on Hofmann 2014

8.6 The Egalitarian Perspective

Fair allocation of benefits between people can be based on the principle of *need*, *merit* or *equality*. In the context of health care allocating benefits according to persons' *needs* is obviously accepted, while *merit* is more controversial. The principle of *equality* is important in just health policy, as displayed in the Nordic countries through equal and universal access to services and (mainly) tax based financing (Vrangbæk et al. 2009). Theoretically, justice requires equality by default if: (a) there are not any relevant distinguishing feature between people that legitimate unequal distribution of advantages and disadvantages or (b) we do not have reliable ways of identifying and measuring the unequal claims people may have (Miller 2017). Certainly, peoples' health conditions lead to legitimate unequal claims for health care services, which is reflected in priority setting criteria like disease severity (associated with medical need) and effects of the treatment (Mobinizadeh et al. 2016). This is not the issue here, as overutilization point towards a low score on priority setting criteria.

We know that radiological services are not distributed equally between groups of people. People living in urban areas with easy access to radiology services are likely to receive more services (Lysdahl and Borretzen 2007; Nixon et al. 2014), whereas e.g. people living in nursing homes are likely to receive less radiology services compared to the general population (Kjelle et al. 2019). Furthermore, the utilization of diagnostic imaging services varies with age, gender, and socioeconomic status (Wang et al. 2008). As these features cause unequal distributions that cannot be explained by differences in medical need, the variation can be judge as unfair, representing a challenge to the principle of equality.

Variation in use is largely associated with overutilization, even if underuse may occur like in the case of nursing home residents receiving less radiological services than the general public despite their higher needs (Kjelle et al. 2019). When overutilization of radiological services is considered to be a bad thing, it is mainly because it results in unnecessary risks from exposure to ionizing radiation and contrast media, false positive results, incidentalomas[1] and overdiagnosis, which in turn can lead to follow up investigations, unnecessary side effects, and (over)treatment. The final outcome may be inflicted harm to the patient in shape of physical and/or metal suffering.

Certainly, people may gain from examinations that were not considered justified in the first place. For now, we limit the good in question to (improved) health outcome. The main advantages used as arguments for a "permissive" practice is the value of detecting diseases at an early (pre-symptomatic) stage. Certainly, true positive findings can be detected incidentally and render possible early access to treatment. One problem with this argument is delimitation: what should be regarded suitable intervals of testing "just in case" of early stage asymptomatic decease? The other unfairness embedded in this argument is that some people will gain from overutilization at the expense of the many who will suffer from increased risks and other disadvantages. Those not receiving too many radiological are most likely better off being spared from the health risks of overutilization. Moreover, there is a strong and partly unwarranted belief in early detection (Hofmann and Skolbekken 2017), that may result in more harm than benefits, i.e. incidental findings of uncertain or low significance, overdiagnosis and overtreatment as mention above.

8.7 The Utilitarian Perspective

Utilitarianism is said to "accommodate and explain much of what we intuitively believe about justice" (Miller 2017) as it is about maximizing the good (Hooker 2016). In this perspective an action is right if it is expected to generate utility, i.e. a higher or equal amount of overall net benefit than other relevant alternatives – all involved parties considered. Still the intuitive understanding can be hard to defend as one of the main objections to utilitarianism, is precisely that it "gives no direct weight to considerations of justice or fairness in the distribution of goods" (Scheffler 1987). Hence, a utilitarian argument for fairness must rest on that fairness will contribute to utility. Preference utilitarianism uses satisfaction of desires as a proxy for utility, and from this point of view it could be argued that providing imaging services in accordance with peoples' desires would justify overutilization. If receiving an examination is considered an intrinsic good, i.e. the value of knowing that you have been investigated with the very best technology, overutilization can be

---

[1] An incidental imaging finding is defined as "an imaging abnormality in a healthy, asymptomatic patient or an imaging abnormality in a symptomatic patient, where the abnormality was not apparently related to the patient's symptoms." (O'Sullivan et al. 2018)

defended. Respecting patients' right to decide does however presuppose that their preferred choices are well informed and sustainable, which may not be the case regarding consequences of too many radiological examinations. It is also commonly claimed that providing imaging services beyond what is strictly medically needed is useful because of its reassuring effect. Utility should be achieved because people feel comforted by an examination "just in case" to confirm their health. However, empirical test of the claim shows that diagnostic tests hardly make any contribution to reassure peoples with various health complaints (van Ravesteijn et al. 2012). Besides, irrelevant radiologic [e.g. degenerative] findings might lead to uncertainty in both GP and patient (Espeland and Baerheim 2003), and reduced well-being. Even if it we could prove the utility of providing services based on the strength of preferences, this can be considered unfair as our expectations are sensitive to whether or not we are used to getting our preferences satisfied (Gandjour and Lauterbach 2003).

Perhaps the most important utilitarian argument against overutilization is the relatively high opportunity costs when material resources (equipment) and personnel are preoccupied with useless (or futile) care. Opportunity costs is the value of the next best choice of utilizing the radiological resources. Within the services, overutilization of imaging can cause queues of patients and displace examinations that would have been more useful (Nuti and Vainieri 2012). "Freeing the resources from low-value care creates new opportunity for redressing underuse within the same budget envelope" (Elshaug et al. 2017). In society at large, the futility and waste associated with overutilization, clearly indicates that higher utility could have been achieved by allocating the resources to other good causes.

From a rule utilitarian perspective justice and fairness are considered rules that when followed will promote overall welfare and happiness. As overutilization of imaging is incompatible with fairness it should be combated from a rule utilitarian point of view.

8.8 The Contractarian Perspective

Contractarianism offers an "understanding of justice by asking the question; what principles to govern institutions, practices and personal behaviour would people choose to adopt if they had to agree on them in advance" (Miller 2017). Such a hypothetical contract based on agreement should ensure that principle chosen would not lead to unacceptable outcomes. In contractarianism the difference principle in Rawls theory of justice states that inequalities should be arranged to the greatest benefit to those least advantaged (ibid). This concerns social and economic inequalities, but here we take the liberty of a broader approach including inequalities in health condition and wellbeing.

Accordingly, the question is who are exposed to overutilization? Some indications are given in the literature about access and drives to services. Patient demands are regarded a major driver of unnecessary imaging (Hendee et al. 2010) (Fig. 8.1), which point to the worried well. However, a vulnerable group of people with high demands are those with chronic muscle and skeletal complaints. For these a referral to imaging services can serve illness legitimisation and the GP have little else to offer (Espeland and Baerheim 2003). Socioeconomic status of patients have been studied and found not to influence the use of scintigraphy, but gender and age do to some extent (Miron et al. 2014). A more direct answer to who receives too much imaging is given in a recent systematic review (Tung et al. 2018). The authors included 20 studies and found that overutilized imaging in emergency departments were greater in older patients, those with higher Injury Severity Scores and those having more comorbid diseases. This means that both people well off and those not so well off are exposed to overutilization. The important point is however that over-utilization seems to add to the burden of those least advantaged.

8.9   Potential Solutions

The problem of overutilization of health care services is vast and complex, which require "levers targeted from the patient level to the government policy making level" (Elshaug et al. 2017). Within the field of medical imaging a number of strate-gies have be suggested to reduce overutilization (Hendee et al. 2010). The tradi-tional approaches include educational strategies towards physicians, patients and the general public (Oren et al. 2019). Educational strategies can focus on under-standing the risks associated with exposing patients to various radiation doses, like the Awareness component in the Triple A approach from the radiation protection bodies (International Agency of Atomic Radiation 2015). Increased awareness about radiation and risks among physicians and patients is assumed to reduce the pressure for redundant examinations (Picano 2004). This strategy seems to be demanding as a number of studies confirm that physicians understanding of radia-tion dose, safety, and potential hazardous effects from imaging remains generally low (Hollingsworth et al. 2019). A strategy focusing on lack of usefulness and risk of harm from incidental and false findings may have higher success, because of the close link to the immediate (expected) outcome of the examination and because these risks are generally easier to grasp. Besides, one could question whether it is fair to kindle peoples' fear of radiation, particularly if the radiation risk is a substi-tute argument for concerns about wasted resources and costs.

The second main strategy is the implementation of appropriateness criteria (Oren et al. 2019), and referral guidelines are developed that can be integrated into elec-tronic referrals or used as a stand-alone web portal (European Society of Radiology 2018). However, it is challenging to make people aware of guidelines in the first place and then to adhere to them (Gransjoen et al. 2018, Tack et al. 2018). It is rec-ognized that the referral decisions can be challenging for the referring physicians, and that they need more support from members of the Department of Radiology (Kruse et al. 2016).

The role of the radiologist in curbing diagnostic waste can be limited to serve as consultant for the referring physician (Otero et al. 2006). A more active approach is to assign radiologists responsibilities for vetting, screening, preauthorizing referrals (Picano et al. 2007). One reason why this approach is not fully utilized (O'Reilly et al. 2009) is the insufficient grounds of the critical assessment, i.e. the lack of clinical information and unclear clinical questions in the referral (Lysdahl et al. 2010).

An alternative approach would be to allow more discretionary power to the radiologist, as argued by Durand et al. (2015): "In the era of value-based care, radiologists must expand beyond their traditional roles as imaging interpreters to become managers of the entire imaging value chain. Ensuring imaging appropriateness is an essential part of that process." One could ask why the referral system require a specific test to be requested, instead of enabling the radiologist to recommend the most appropriate diagnostic test in the clinical situation (Kenny and Pacey 2005). Radiographers can also contribute to justified examinations by evaluating the amount and quality of information in the referrals (Vom and Williams 2017), by providing supplementary information (Hannah and McConnell 2009), and by authorizing referrals according to guidelines (Matthews and Brennan 2008). The advantage of increasing the engagement of radiologist and radiographer to combat overutilization is first and foremost that they are in a better position of keeping updated about appropriate procedures. They may also be less responsive to patient demands. Finally, it can be argued that is fair to allow them more influence as they are ultimately responsible for the services they provide, and excessive utilization and unnecessary examinations represents a practical and moral challenge in their daily work (Gottlieb 2005; Lewis 2002; Wilner 2007).

More attention should also be paid to biases, inclinations, and imperatives in handling technology. A wide range of irrational (psychological and emotional) mechanisms have been identified in assessing and implementing technologies (Hofmann 2019). Paying attention to such mechanisms is crucial when addressing overutilization of imaging. In addition to strategies towards the professionals, more attention should be paid to organizational aspects like, ownership of equipment (Hong et al. 2017) and payment scheme (Iversen and Mokienko 2016). Fortunately, the international Choosing Wisely campaign (Levinson et al. 2015) together with other measures to reduce overuse have shown that it is possible to address overutilization of radiological services.

8.10 Conclusion

We have tried to show that overutilization may be difficult to define and measure, and that it has a wide range of drivers. Overutilization is morally problematic, and incompatible with fairness across three conceptions of the term: because of the arbitrary distribution of benefits and risk between people with equal medical needs (egalitarian perspective), the distribution of services that will not maximise utility (utilitarian perspective), and overutilization does not benefit those least advantaged (contractarian). While there is a wide range of suggested measures to halt or reduce overutilization, there are no easy solutions to a serious problem to modern health care. Strategies are needed at political, organisational and professional level, where interdisciplinary efforts are needed.

References

Abrams, H.L. 1979. The overutilization of X-rays. *New England Journal of Medicine* 300 (21): 1213–1216.

Adams, S.J., R. Rakheja, R. Bryce, and P.S. Babyn. 2018. Incidence and economic impact of incidental findings on (18)F-FDG PET/CT imaging. *Canadian Association of Radiologists Journal* 69 (1): 63–70. https://doi.org/10.1016/j.carj.2017.08.001.

Almén, A., W. Leitz, and S. Richter. 2009. *National Survey on justification of CT-examination in Sweden. Rapport number 2009:03.* Stockholm: Swedish Radiation Safety Authority.

Blachar, A., S. Tal, A. Mandel, I. Novikov, G. Polliack, J. Sosna, Y. Freedman, L. Copel, and J. Shemer. 2006. Preauthorization of CT and MRI examinations: Assessment of a managed care preauthorization program based on the ACR Appropriateness Criteria and the Royal College of Radiology guidelines. *Journal of the American College of Radiology* 3 (11): 851–859. https://doi.org/10.1016/j.jacr.2006.04.005.

Clement, C.H., and H. Ogino. 2018. ICRP publication 138: Ethical foundations of the system of radiological protection. *Annals of the ICRP* 47 (1): 1–65. https://doi.org/10.1177/0146645317746010.

Durand, D.J., G. McGinty, and R. Duszak Jr. 2015. From gatekeeper to Steward: The evolving concept of radiologist accountability for imaging utilization. *Journal of the American College of Radiology* 12 (12 Pt B): 1446–1448. https://doi.org/10.1016/j.jacr.2015.06.031.

Elshaug, A.G., M.B. Rosenthal, J.N. Lavis, S. Brownlee, H. Schmidt, S. Nagpal, P. Littlejohns, D. Srivastava, S. Tunis, and V. Saini. 2017. Levers for addressing medical underuse and overuse: Achieving high-value health care. *Lancet* 390 (10090): 191–202. https://doi.org/10.1016/S0140-6736(16)32586-7.

Espeland, A., and A. Baerheim. 2003. Factors affecting general practitioners' decisions about plain radiography for back pain: Implications for classification of guideline barriers--a qualitative study. *BMC Health Services Research* 3 (1): 8.

European Society of Radiology. 2018. *ESR iGuide – Clinical decision support using European imaging referral guidelines.* Vienna: European Society of Radiology.

Gandjour, A., and K.W. Lauterbach. 2003. Utilitarian theories reconsidered: Common misconceptions, more recent developments, and health policy implications. *Health Care Analysis* 11 (3): 229–244.

Gottlieb, R.H. 2005. Imaging for whom: Patient or physician? *AJR. American Journal of Roentgenology* 185 (6): 1399–1403.

Gransjoen, A.M., S. Wiig, K.B. Lysdahl, and B.M. Hofmann. 2018. Barriers and facilitators for guideline adherence in diagnostic imaging: An explorative study of GPs' and radiologists' perspectives. *BMC Health Services Research* 18 (1): 556. https://doi.org/10.1186/s12913-018-3372-7.

Gunderman, R.B. 2005. The medical community's changing vision of the patient: The importance of radiology. *Radiology* 234 (2): 339–342.

Hall, F.M. 1976. Overutilization of radiological examinations. *Radiology* 120 (2): 443–448.

Hannah, S., and J. McConnell. 2009. Serratia marcescens: A case history to illustrate the value of radiographer history taking in the face of poor health professional communication. *Radiography* 15 (4): e34–e43. https://doi.org/10.1016/j.radi.2009.03.005.

Hendee, W.R., G.J. Becker, J.P. Borgstede, J. Bosma, W.J. Casarella, B.A. Erickson, C.D. Maynard, J.H. Thrall, and P.E. Wallner. 2010. Addressing overutilization in medical imaging. *Radiology* 257 (1): 240–245. https://doi.org/10.1148/radiol.10100063.

Hofmann, B. 2010. Too much of a good thing is wonderful? A conceptual analysis of excessive examinations and diagnostic futility in diagnostic radiology. *Medicine, Health Care, and Philosophy* 13 (2): 139–148. https://doi.org/10.1007/s11019-010-9233-8.

———. 2014. Diagnosing overdiagnosis. *European Journal of Epidemiology* 29: 599–604. https://doi.org/10.1007/s10654-014-9920-5.

———. 2019. Biases and imperatives in handling medical technology. *Health Policy and Technology* 8 (4): 377–385. https://doi.org/10.1016/j.hlpt.2019.10.005.

Hofmann, B., and J.-A. Skolbekken. 2017. Surge in publications on early detection. *BMJ* 357: j2102. https://doi.org/10.1136/bmj.j2102.

Hollingsworth, T.D., R. Duszak Jr., A. Vijayasarathi, R.B. Gelbard, and M.E. Mullins. 2019. Trainee knowledge of imaging appropriateness and safety: Results of a series of surveys from a large academic medical center. *Current Problems in Diagnostic Radiology* 48 (1): 17–21. https://doi.org/10.1067/j.cpradiol.2017.10.007.

Hong, A.S., D. Ross-Degnan, F. Zhang, and J.F. Wharam. 2017. Clinician-level predictors for ordering low-value imaging. *JAMA Internal Medicine* 177 (11): 1577–1585. https://doi.org/10.1001/jamainternmed.2017.4888.

Hooker, B. 2016. *Rule consequentialism. The Stanford encyclopedia of philosophy.* https://plato.stanford.edu/archives/win2016/entries/consequentialism-rule/.

International Agency of Atomic Radiation. 2015. *Radiation protection in medicine: Setting the scene for the next decade: Proceedings of an International Conference, Bonn, 3–7 December 2012.* Vienna: IAEA Proceedings Series. ISSN 0074–1884.

Iversen, T., and A. Mokienko. 2016. Supplementing gatekeeping with a revenue scheme for secondary care providers. *International Journal of Health Economics and Management* 16 (3): 247–267. https://doi.org/10.1007/s10754-016-9188-2.

Kenny, L.M., and F. Pacey. 2005. The perils of the "remote" radiologist. *Medical Journal of Australia* 183 (11–12): 630–619.

Kevles, B.H. 1997. *Naked to the bone. Medical imaging in the twentieth century.* New Bruswick: Rutgers University Press. Reprint, On Request.

Kjelle, Elin, Kristin Bakke Lysdahl, and Hilde Merete Olerud. 2019. Impact of mobile radiography services in nursing homes on the utilisation of diagnostic imaging procedures. *BMC Health Services Research* 19 (1): 428. https://doi.org/10.1186/s12913-019-4276-x.

Koutalonis, M., and J. Horrocks. 2012. Justification in clinical radiological practice: A survey among staff of five London hospitals. *Radiation Protection Dosimetry* 149 (2): 124–137. https://doi.org/10.1093/rpd/ncr211.

Kruse, J., N. Lehto, K. Riklund, Y. Tegner, and A. Engstrom. 2016. Scrutinized with inadequate control and support: Interns' experiences communicating with and writing referrals to hospital radiology departments – A qualitative study. *Radiography* 22 (4): 313–318. https://doi.org/10.1016/j.radi.2016.04.004.

Lalumera, E., S. Fanti, and G. Boniolo. 2019. Reliability of molucular imanign diagnostics. *Synthese.* https://doi.org/10.1007/s11229-019-02419-y.

Lehnert, B.E., and R.L. Bree. 2010. Analysis of appropriateness of outpatient CT and MRI referred from primary care clinics at an academic medical center: How critical is the necd for improved decision support? *Journal of the American College of Radiology* 7 (3): 192–197. https://doi.org/10.1016/j.jacr.2009.11.010.

Levinson, W., M. Kallewaard, R.S. Bhatia, D. Wolfson, S. Shortt, and E.A. Kerr. 2015. 'Choosing Wisely': A growing international campaign. *BMJ Quality and Safety* 24 (2): 167–174. https://doi.org/10.1136/bmjqs-2014-003821.

Lewis, S. 2002. Reflection and identification of ethical issues in Australian radiography. *The Radiographer* 49: 151–156.

Lysdahl, K.B., and I. Borretzen. 2007. Geographical variation in radiological services: A nation-wide survey. *BMC Health Services Research* 7: 21. https://doi.org/10.1186/1472-6963-7-21.

Lysdahl, K.B., B.M. Hofmann, and A. Espeland. 2010. Radiologists' responses to inadequate referrals. *European Radiology* 20 (5): 1227–1233. https://doi.org/10.1007/s00330-009-1640-y.

Matthews, K., and P.C. Brennan. 2008. Justification of x-ray examinations: General principles and an Irish perspective. *Radiography* 14 (4): 349–355.

McClenahan, J.L. 1970. Wasted x-rays. *Radiology* 96 (2): 453–458.

Miller, D. 2017. *Justice, the Stanford encyclopedia of philosophy.* https://plato.stanford.edu/archives/fall2017/entries/justice/.

Miron, S.D., M. Gutu, and V. Astarastoae. 2014. Is it enough scintigraphy for everyone? A cross-sectional analysis regarding the impact of justice in the distribution of health care resources. *Revista Medico-Chirurgicala A Societatii de Medici si Naturalisti din Iasi* 118 (4): 1094–1100.

Mobinizadeh, M., P. Raeissi, A.A. Nasiripour, A. Olyaeemanesh, and S.J. Tabibi. 2016. The health systems' priority setting criteria for selecting health technologies: A systematic review of the current evidence. *Medical Journal of the Islamic Republic of Iran* 30: 329.

Nixon, G., A. Samaranayaka, B. de Graaf, R. McKechnie, K. Blattner, and S. Dovey. 2014. Geographic disparities in the utilisation of computed tomography scanning services in southern New Zealand. *Health Policy* 118 (2): 222–228. https://doi.org/10.1016/j.healthpol.2014.05.002.

Nuti, S., and M. Vainieri. 2012. Managing waiting times in diagnostic medical imaging. *BMJ Open* 2 (6): e001255. https://doi.org/10.1136/bmjopen-2012-001255.

O'Reilly, G., E. Gruppetta, S. Christofides, A. Schreiner-Karoussou, and A. Dowling. 2009. Rapporteurs' report: Workshop on ethical issues in diagnostic radiology. *Radiation Protection Dosimetry* 135 (2): 122–127.

O'Sullivan, J.W., T. Muntinga, S. Grigg, and J.P.A. Ioannidis. 2018. Prevalence and outcomes of incidental imaging findings: Umbrella review. *BMJ* 361: k2387. https://doi.org/10.1136/bmj.k2387.

Oren, O., E. Kebebew, and J.P.A. Ioannidis. 2019. Curbing unnecessary and wasted diagnostic imaging. *Journal of the American Medical Association* 321: 245. https://doi.org/10.1001/jama.2018.20295.

Otero, H.J., S. Ondategui-Parra, E.M. Nathanson, S.M. Erturk, and P.R. Ros. 2006. Utilization management in radiology: Basic concepts and applications. *Journal of the American College of Radiology* 3 (5): 351–357. https://doi.org/10.1016/j.jacr.2006.01.006.

Picano, E. 2004. Sustainability of medical imaging. *BMJ* 328 (7439): 578–580.

Picano, E., E. Pasanisi, J. Brown, and T.H. Marwick. 2007. A gatekeeper for the gatekeeper: Inappropriate referrals to stress echocardiography. *American Heart Journal* 154 (2): 285–290. https://doi.org/10.1016/j.ahj.2007.04.032.

Rawle, M., and A. Pighills. 2018. Prevalence of unjustified emergency department x-ray examination referrals performed in a regional Queensland hospital: A pilot study. *Journal of Medical Radiation Sciences* 65 (3): 184–191. https://doi.org/10.1002/jmrs.287.

Saini, V., S. Garcia-Armesto, D. Klemperer, V. Paris, A.G. Elshaug, S. Brownlee, J.P.A. Ioannidis, and E.S. Fisher. 2017. Drivers of poor medical care. *Lancet* 390 (10090): 178–190. https://doi.org/10.1016/S0140-6736(16)30947-3.

Scheffler, Samuel. 1987. *Consequentialism and its critics.* Oxford: Oxford University Press. Reprint, Not in File.

Simpson, G., and G.S. Hartrick. 2007. Use of thoracic computed tomography by general practitioners. *Medical Journal of Australia* 187 (1): 43–46.

Tack, D., F. Louage, A. Van Muylem, N. Howarth, and P.A. Gevenois. 2018. Radiation protection: Factors influencing compliance to referral guidelines in minor chest trauma. *European Radiology* 28 (4): 1420–1426. https://doi.org/10.1007/s00330-017-5093-4.

Tahvonen, P., H. Oikarinen, E. Niinimaki, E. Liukkonen, S. Mattila, and O. Tervonen. 2017. Justification and active guideline implementation for spine radiography referrals in primary care. *Acta Radiologica* 58 (5): 586–592. https://doi.org/10.1177/0284185116661879.

Tung, M., R. Sharma, J.S. Hinson, S. Nothelle, J. Pannikottu, and J.B. Segal. 2018. Factors associated with imaging overuse in the emergency department: A systematic review. *The American Journal of Emergency Medicine* 36 (2): 301–309. https://doi.org/10.1016/j.ajem.2017.10.049.

van Ravesteijn, H., I. van Dijk, D. Darmon, F. van de Laar, P. Lucassen, T.O. Hartman, C. van Weel, and A. Speckens. 2012. The reassuring value of diagnostic tests: A systematic review. *Patient Education and Counseling* 86 (1): 3–8. https://doi.org/10.1016/j.pec.2011.02.003.

Vom, J., and I. Williams. 2017. Justification of radiographic examinations: What are the key issues? *Journal of Medical Radiation Sciences* 11: 11. https://doi.org/10.1002/jmrs.211.

Vrangbæk, Karsten, Richard B. Saltman, and Jon Magnussen. 2009. *Nordic health care systems: Recent reforms and current policy challenges, European observatory on health systems and policies series.* Maidenhead: McGraw-Hill/Open University Press.

Wang, L., J.X. Nie, C.S. Tracy, R. Moineddin, and R.E. Upshur. 2008. Utilization patterns of diagnostic imaging across the late life course: A population-based study in Ontario, Canada. *International Journal of Technology Assessment in Health Care* 24 (4): 384–390. https://doi.org/10.1017/s0266462308080501.

Wilner, E.M. 2007. Are we really practicing medicine today? *Radiology* 245 (2): 330.

Chapter 9
The Philosophical and Ethical Issues Facing Imaging Professionals When Communicating Diagnostic Imaging Results to Oncologic Patients

Laetitia Marcucci and David Taïeb

Abstract Over the last few decades, medical imaging has gained an increasing importance in oncology at *every step* along *the cancer care* pathway (e.g., detection, staging, post-treatment assessment, detection of recurrence). With the explosion of information available on the internet and shared decision-making, the patients are often aware that imaging results can have a major impact on their care programme. Therefore, they are particularly keen on enquiring about the results as soon as the examination has been completed. The article proposes an analysis of the philosophical and ethical aspects involved in communicating bad news following imaging examinations of oncologic patients, with special emphasis on nuclear imaging.

Keywords Oncology · Imaging · Ethics

Discussion and conclusions: While communicating bad news in a sympathetic way is an essential ability for medical professionals, there is a paucity of educational curricula on interpersonal and communication skills in imaging. Research is still required to determine ideal methods for educating senior-level physicians and residents on communicating diagnostic imaging results. Role-play scenarios could represent an appropriate method to achieve this goal by taking into account the context

L. Marcucci
ADES (UMR 7268), Aix-Marseille University, Marseille, France

CRHI (EA 4318), Université Côte d'Azur, Nice, France

Espace de Réflexion Éthique Régional PACA-Corse, Nice et Marseille, France
e-mail: laetitia.marcucci@univ-amu.fr; laetitia.marcucci@univ-cotedazur.fr

D. Taïeb (✉)
Department of Nuclear Medicine, La Timone University Hospital, CERIMED,
Aix-Marseille University, Marseille, France
e-mail: david.taieb@ap-hm.fr

© The Author(s), under exclusive license to Springer Nature
Switzerland AG 2020
E. Lalumera, S. Fanti (eds.), *Philosophy of Advanced Medical Imaging*,
SpringerBriefs in Ethics, https://doi.org/10.1007/978-3-030-61412-6_9

of respecting the patients' right to decide whether they wish to receive such information and their right to their own autonomy, with personalised approaches to better adapt to their capacity and vulnerability.

Training in the breaking of bad news, with the required communication skills, is currently a very small part of medical education, more focused on technical know-how than on soft skills. The context of medical imaging related to medical oncology is a very specific and topical point. Owing to the shock and the power of images in relation to cultural mindsets, these examinations are awaited but much dreaded by patients. Regardless of their predictive value, images raise questions, and the choice of words is very important as they will be carefully weighed up as what they may or may not mean. In addition to honestly providing the purely medical information in an understandable way, the physician must consider, from an ethical point of view, the emotional impact on the patient. In addition, with multiple stakeholders around the patient, informational and communicational issues have many levels and dimensions. The role played by the medical imagery specialist in relation to oncology has thus to be clarified in the interest of the patient. Little research has been done on this situation which is a common occurrence for nuclear physicians. Building on a philosophical and applied ethical approach, the aim of this paper is to identify the ethical issues at stake, to show the need for ethical guidelines in the context of medical imaging daily practice, and finally to suggest appropriate standards. While observing the rules of professional practice, informational and communicational risks are connected with the need to respect the patient, taking into account both their capacity and vulnerability. First, ethical questions will be considered in the light of the specific medical issues and the context of imaging cancer patients. Then, informational and communicational issues must be contrasted with the vulnerability of the patients concerned, their need for autonomy to be respected and perhaps to be empowered in uncertain environments. Finally, on the basis of a typology of situations, we will offer guidelines for implementing ethical practices and policies for accompanying these processes.

9.1 Context and Main Issues

9.1.1 The Concepts of Disease and Health

Illness makes us experience finitude. Indeed, beyond the materiality of the body, illness is an embodied experience of the violence of life (Marin 2008a, b). It upsets the balance of good health that is characterised by simple daily actions and routines, and reduces confidence in everyday habits, on which the sense of one's own identity is often built (Marin 2014). What is most unsettling is that life threatening diseases affect all aspects of daily life, starting with the individual perception of what constitutes personal identity. In this way, in the etymological meaning of the word, illness can be considered as a *catastrophic* experience (Marin 2014). What is more, especially when the disease is serious or chronic, it impacts all dimensions of the individual, leading to a "slow social death" (Marin 2014).

How can someone know that they are sick? The need for clear differentiation between the normal or pathological is deceived by ordinary experience and by clinical findings. Disease corresponds to an inner state that is specific to the person in their singularity and cannot be related to a general extrinsic norm (Canguilhem 1966). Moreover, the task of isolating biomedical causes of a patient's suffering, in other words the medical understanding of illness, differs sharply from the understanding of the patients' experience of it. The former involves clinical observations and (non-)invasive examinations while the latter is essentially an existential experience.

In fact, when it occurs, disease reshapes our mental states, and misrepresentations of good health are unmasked. The experience of illness reminds us of the fragility of human life and our vulnerability to bodily changes that affect us. As V. Jankelevitch points out in his philosophical essay *Death* (Jankelevitch 1966), according to the ancient Latin saying, *Mors certa, hora incerta*. We do not know the hour of our death, although we can be sure that this moment will occur. Good health leaves the certainty of the end floating. Moreover, regardless of disease, a multiplicity of events might be fatal. The lack of certainty about the precise moment and circumstances of death seem to be a kind of indeterminacy which reopens the field of possibilities at the very core of human existence. In the case of diagnosis, particularly when the possibility of cancer is mentioned, the expectation of the end of life becomes more present and ever more pressing, even though treatments may provide remissions, delaying the imminence of *incerta hora* (Jankelevitch 1966).

From a medical point of view, disease does not always foreshadow death. But, in our societies, cancer is still too often associated with a fatal outcome, as if those who have it should be regarded as doomed by fate to a shorter run, and to die in great suffering. For these reasons, whether a prognosis is confirmed or invalidated, the context of the diagnosis announcement is emotionally highly charged. Evidence based medicine relies on technical examinations and risk assessment. Although it may suggest that uncertainty is set aside, physicians' reasoning is based on decision trees and probability calculations, which does not exclude the risk of error, correlated to the current state of knowledge and technological limits. In this context, patients experience a kind of squared uncertainty which deserves an intensified focus.

We shall now examine the specific context of nuclear imaging in oncology.

9.1.2 The Patient-Nuclear Physician Relationship

Nuclear (molecular) imaging and more specifically Positron Emission Tomography – Computed Tomography (PET/CT) imaging plays a central role in oncology by allowing *in vivo* visualization of molecular dysregulation as well as over-expression of certain cell membrane transporters, receptors or tumour antigens. This is made possible through the availability of a wide diversity of radiopharmaceuticals (tracers). Among these tracers, F-18 fluorodeoxyglucose (an 18F-labeled glucose analog, also called FDG) has a major role at various steps of cancer management: staging malignancy, evaluating tumour response to treatment, evaluating indeterminate masses discovered on CT, MRI and US.

After PET/CT examination, nuclear physicians should depict all uptake foci with a precise conclusion regarding their nature and include these findings in a specific clinical trial. The added value of molecular imaging over classic radiological imaging relies on the use of various radiopharmaceuticals specific to certain situations (i.e., neuroendocrine malignancies) and these are avidly taken up by tumours. The high tumour-to-background uptake ratio is optimal for tumour detection (sensitivity), and associated with a high positive predictive value avoiding the elevated rate of false positive results generally associated with very sensitive anatomic imaging modalities. Nowadays, PET/CT can be performed in many institutions, including academic and private ones. Expert recommendations for the use of PET/CT imaging in oncology have been published by various learned societes and provide detailed information regarding performance in various clinical scenarios. (Salaün et al. 2020). The value of PET/CT is largely dependent on the size, origin and aggressive behaviour of the tumour. For example, FDG-PET/CT has high sensitivity (around 95%) for the diagnosis of solid pulmonary nodules ≥ 8 mm. Nuclear physicians are also aware that some inflammatory or infectious lesions (tuberculosis, sarcoidosis and histoplasmosis) may give false-positive results. By contrast, FDG-PET/CT has low sensitivity and specificity for informing on the malignancy of a breast lesion.

PET/CT reports should include the following information: (1) Confirm diagnosis of cancer or persistence/recurrence in doubtful situations; (2) Evaluate locoregional extension, of the disease which, together with anatomic imaging, can select candidates for potential focused therapeutic intervention (surgery, interventional radiology, radiotherapy); (3) Rule out or detect potential metastases in distant organs; (4) Predict aggressiveness via quantitative imaging biomarkers.

The patients know that PET scans have a major impact on the decision-making process. Furthermore, patients tend to find imaging reports more objective than other medical test results, and they perceive them as the most conclusive evidence for their condition. Hence, they are particularly keen on enquiring about the results on the day of the PET procedure itself.

However, the patient-nuclear physician relationship is unique for many reasons. After the nuclear medicine imaging, the patient-physician encounter is often short due to radioprotection and/or organizational constraints. The nuclear physician is confronted with challenging situations in which they are expected to deliver diagnostic results, without prior understanding of the emotional status or psychological backgrounds of patients. The patient is often unknown to the nuclear physician due to limited scheduled follow-up. Finally, the nuclear physician may be disconnected from the global therapeutic strategy, for instance in the case where the situation is controlled by the referring specialist team from another institution (Gonzalez et al. 2018a).

9.1.3 The Power of Medical Images

While the sociological and psychological dimensions correlated to patients' expectations regarding nuclear examinations could be identified by the use of criteria such as sex, age, education, income, cultural background, etc., from an anthropological, philosophical and ethical point of view, the focus point is still the shock and power of images, which are quite often symbolically and emotionally overloaded. From an epistemological point of view, even if the image can also sometimes be an obstacle to rational understanding, the imaged representation that promotes the perception of reality, in particular when it improves on the eye's unaided performance, is part of the scientific process that determines facts, additionally "scientific rationality is often the ally of imagination" (Wunenburger 1997). However, images reign supreme in our occidental societies of appearances. Special attention given to images is strengthened by the multiplication of screens and associated technologies (PET/CT imaging, MRI, ultrasound images...), which provide numerical body modelling and data schematizations, to such an extent that the risk of being fascinated by them, is not to be underestimated (Joyce 2008; Van Dijk 2005). The quality of the images is not unrelated to the powers of science, and the effects they have on both the expert and the person receiving care cannot be ignored (Wunenburger 1997).

Nevertheless, images are not mere raw data, but on the contrary reconstructions of a complex reality both shown and hidden, because images have something to do with the invisible (Masson 2007). Moreover, pictures are representations of sensitive data, which are part of an inherently dynamic, uncertain and evolving process (Delehanty 2010). While images are not reality, they pave the way to belief and over-confidence in their power, and correlatively, to mismatched expectations and excessive hopes. At the same time, they determine attitudes towards knowledge and expertise, which must be taken into account. Owing to the naïve belief in pictorial evidence, the main misinterpretation of the role of images may be reinforced by the patient's stress surrounding nuclear examinations. They risk overestimating the importance of images and the crucial part played in reading them during diagnosis. So, they might consider the images to be instantaneous revelations of "Truth". However, the interpretation process is very complex and the likelihood of error in the interpretation of medical images is not negligible (Krupinski 2010). It is considered here that truth is where the concept corresponds to reality, and thus the very possibility of doubting, risks being excluded from the process (Potier 2007).

There are many aspects which may lead a patient to feel lost in this excessively technical and stressful context: (1) The interpretation of images requires a mastery of complex codes because it is necessary to connect, combine and interpret several levels of understanding; (2) The cross-connections with the real world that advanced virtual imaging techniques provide are numerous and produce much additional data; (3) Multi-omics approaches multiply the levels of complexity (Gillies et al. 2015). Those who do not have a significant scientific or medical culture i.e. the vast majority of patients (Potier 2007), are likely to be seduced by an over-simplification of the image and have faith in that rather than medical expertise which honestly reveals the real uncertainty surrounding many cases. The power and shock of refined images can thus only be strengthened, all the more so since the physical body imaged is first and foremost for the patient his or her living body, whereas for the radiologist the physical body is what he works with primarily through examinations (Estival 2010). *A minima*, the body revealed by imaging techniques is a body-object that does not fail to raise issues related to identity, self-recognition, even though personal identity cannot be reduced to scientific objectification, as philosophers and psychologists have shown (Marin 2008a, b, 2014; Potier 2012).

So, the techniques constitute an intermediate space between patients and physicians and therefore the images can prevent or facilitate adherence to the treatment. It all depends on the moment when the medical imaging act is performed and the place it will take in the history of the patients and their illness. The images, and their manner of presentation as well as what they represent, crystallise expectations and questions in particularly charged situations such as those experienced in oncology. If we continue in the vein of mental representations on the one hand, and of metaphysical expectations and needs on the other hand, "the statement of the diagnosis is often understood as prognosis and therefore, let us be clear, as destiny" (Harrus-Révidi 2008). In the face of the uncertainty of the *hora*, to escape the certainty of dying, *mors certa*, that becomes more tangible, the patient may be tempted to rely entirely on the "blind authority of the image" that precedes the words, as if in a modern ordeal; hence the importance of listening and speaking to the doctor, in order to dispel possible illusions and to conduct the care process rationally and humanely (Ricœur 1990; Assoun 2009).

All these elements can explain the discrepancy between the actual prognosis and the impact of the announcement on people's lives, and these two must be distinguished. To the sensitivity to negative information on the patient side, it is necessary to respond with increased attention on how to relay information, not only to the speech that carries the information but also to the need for concern, care and solicitude, while ontological vulnerabilities are prevalent.

9.2 Ethical Issues and Current Practices

9.2.1 Shared Ethical Principles

In the case of medical imaging, professional practices have evolved towards the multi-disciplinary, often with a confrontation between logic and expertise. It is more than ever necessary to cross-reference approaches, but several risks have already been identified with regard to communicating imaging test results to patients, especially when the relational aspect, which involves changes in professional practices, are not really considered, and this raises ethical issues (Béranger and Le Coz 2012). The need recognised in much Western legislation for clear, fair and appropriate information derives from the application of the main ethical principles set out at the end of the Second World War, based on the Nuremberg Code (The Nuremberg Code 1947), the first medical deontology code (Weindling 2001), and the major international texts and treaties, such as the 1948 Universal Declaration of Human Rights (Kemp and Rendtorff 2000; Kemp et al. 2000). These ethical guidelines emphasise the dignity and respect of the human person, the inviolability of the human body, the importance of obtaining informed consent in biomedical research, and the right to withdraw (World Medical Association 2013; Centre d'études et de recherche sanitaire et médico-sociale de Poitiers 1990). However, serious illness, from the point of view of medical data, or considered as such from the point of view of social and individual representations, produces increased vulnerability among people who are confronted by it. People suffering disease, regardless of the techniques used to cure it, can be helped or hindered in their existentially understood journey and their emotional, psychological and social need. Whether or not the disease can finally be cured, whether or not there are delays to be obtained with regard to the time of death, *mors certa, hora incerta*, the time of life remains to be lived because we are, in all cases, "alive until death" (Ricœur 2007; Jankelevitch 1966).

As a result of the recommendations for good practice, attitudes are changing, and the focus is increasingly on the patient. That the patient can be an actor in their health implies that they are really considered as an autonomous subject, capable of understanding and deciding for themselves, and therefore can participate in the cure and care that will be provided to them. The paternalistic paradigm that was widely criticised by Beauchamp and Childress in their book entitled *Principles of Biomedical Ethics* (Beauchamp and Childress 1979) is increasingly disregarded, in favour of the paradigm of patient autonomy or even of their *empowerment*. In this context, the principle of beneficence (*bene facere*), includes both the provision of beneficial effects (*facere bonum*) to the patients, and the patient's understanding and acceptation that the element, currently under discussion, of the care programme is beneficial. The hippocratic principle *primum non nocere*, the principle of "non-maleficence", continues to guide ethical reflection. Whether it's good or bad, how news is announced and perceived, especially when the situation is emotionally charged, may, in extreme cases, help the patient's wellbeing, even when there is no hope of a cure. On the other hand, it could be perceived as a death sentence which closes the field of possibilities, and may finally result in refusal, denial or even the patients' abandonment of their care project. News delivered with tact and consideration for the person and their moral, psychological and physical integrity can reveal unsuspected resources to them.

But how to deliver quality information, adapted to the patients' clinical context, but also to their capacities of understanding, individual preferences, ways of seeing life, and aspirations? What is at stake here is the recognition of the patient, as an individual, in the intersubjective relationship that the practitioner establishes with them (Ricœur 2004). Thanks to this relationship, care becomes a genuine gift. Moreover, investing in quality communication leads to the fourth guiding principle, namely justice, since it potentially represents both an ethical and an economic gain, in so far as positive benefits can be expected for the patient. Thus, in medical terms, good treatment compliance and adhesion to the care project is one potential out-come, whereas the necessity of common values in health care is central to this pro-cess. Indeed, the point is to consider singular individuals, to show them the respect they deserve, allowing for their ontological vulnerabilities, by being mindful of what the philosopher E. Levinas called their "faces", because face-to-face encoun-ters entail high responsibilities and duties for individuals (Levinas 1984).

Although very widely applied in care institutions, the Principlism based approach has been criticised (Walker 2009) as lacking universality and context. It should be highlighted that if "some moral rules are universally shared", nevertheless some decision criteria must be adjusted to specific contexts, because "some ethical responses are very dependent on context" (Tassy et al. 2008). Thus, in daily medical practice, nuclear physicians are facing the need to provide quality information. Moreover, ethical concern for justice requires that stakeholders treat each as a unique case whilst betraying "the rule of action" as little as possible, that is what Paul Ricœur calls "practical wisdom" or "ethical cautiousness", in line with Aristotelian phronesis (Ricœur 1990, 1995).

9.2.2   Ethics in Communication

Medical daily practice has moved away from a one-to-one situation towards a model of collegiality and shared decision-making. In care protocols, how should room be made for discourse, that of both the patient and their doctors and specifically here, for conversations with the nuclear physician? The right balance needs to be estab-lished between the several interlocutors involved. The radiologist must preserve the trust previously established with other physicians while also being careful to main-tain the patient's relationships with the entire medical team. They must also respect the requirements for quality and accuracy of information.

Moreover, speech and discourse have meaning for the human world (Gusdorf 1952). Speech is not only a vector of information and communication. It is much more. In intersubjectivity, the fundamental, ontological level of our existence is involved. This is what brings the speaker out of their isolation. People speak with the body (non-verbal language), with words (verbal language), but also with ail-ments and symptoms, if we refer to psychoanalytic theory. The word is singular because it is carried by subjects, themselves carriers of complex intentions and meanings, which thus give meaning to the world in order to be able to inhabit it. The word, which is at the heart of intersubjective and interpersonal relationships, is cre-ative: it can both liberate and/or alienate us according to the use we make of it.

Speech and discourse imply the building of communication and the consistency of information, which relies on "shaping ideas for a briefing" (Terrou 1962), because communication is an ongoing process of information sharing, which involves sig-nals and channels. In other words, "communication is an act and information is its product", and it requires the development of strategies (Escarpit 1991). First, a con-tact must be established for the communication to take place. The modalities of transmission and relationship are not neutral to the meaning produced and received. There is nothing more volatile and perishable than information: "Not only does the relevant information vary from one individual to another, but it varies for each individual as circumstances change" (Bougnoux 2009). When speech no longer connects, fails to create links between or make sense to people, this leads to situations of incommunicability and loss of information (fading). In the context of the study of philosophical and ethical issues for imaging professionals, the point is the connection of speech and discourse with the world of medical technology, since according to Albert Camus, "misnaming an object is adding to the misfortune of the world". This means respecting individual sensitivities. Thus, in complex care settings and when there is uncertainty about the outcome, ethical concern for others involves thinking, not only about the choice of words, but also about appropriate attitudes.

The current practice of breaking bad news among radiologists and nuclear physicians is the following. Delivering imaging results to cancer patients is traditionally performed by the oncologists. However, the patients are particularly keen on enquiring about the results on the day of the PET procedure itself. Therefore, the daily practice of nuclear physicians as radiologists often include routine communication of imaging results directly to oncologic patients. There is increasing interest in expanding direct communication throughout nuclear medicine and radiology. This duty can be shared by senior-level physicians or even residents. A recent study has shown that a large majority of radiology residents have communicated test results to patients, yet 83.6% described no training in communicating such results to patients. A large majority of residents expressed interest in obtaining additional communication training (Narayan et al. 2018). It is mainly the public universitary hospitals that are concerned with the daily announcement of bad news.

As for the French context, since 2002, with the Kouchner law on the rights of patients, with emphasis placed on the delivery of information and its quality, the applicable legal framework has been evolving in favour of the increasing autonomy of patients. This marks an end to the paternalistic approach of medicine, and ensures the raising of awareness of their rights for the patients themselves, which means they become responsible actors, with whom medical teams must work hand in hand. Thus, specific announcement protocols have been introduced in some hospitals, especially for breast cancers. However, they are not widespread, whatever the circumstances and type of cancer. Delivering imaging results to cancer patients is an important aspect of their overall management. This duty is shared by all healthcare providers and could be considered as a good medical practice. However, there are currently no guidelines or legislation addressing the content and magnitude of information to be delivered to patients.

A recently performed French survey revealed a wide heterogeneity of practices in nuclear medicine departments, for: (1) pre and/or post PET consultations for patients: systematic for 56%, adapted on a case-to-case basis for 35%, and never for 9% of the respondents; (2) oral communication of results to patients: systematic for 13%, adapted on a case-to-case basis for 63%, and never for 24% of the respondents. Working in a private centre, presence of pre-PET consultations, and having more years of experience in nuclear medicine were significantly associated with a greater tendency to orally communicate PET results (Gonzalez et al. 2018b). Many respondents declared that they were very uncomfortable about the disclosure of results, mainly due to lack of clear and specific recommendations and training dedicated to the breaking of bad news.

Although many actors are involved, nuclear physicians play a central role in the information cycle. They must deal with patients with whom they may not be familiar. When it comes to delivering such technical medical information, based on data that is in some respects volatile and ambiguous, there is no substitute for human contact. Of course, physicians must take into account the different types of information to be provided and the time periods specific to them, with regard to the question of mastering therapeutic issues and depending on the context. Ethics in communication here requires careful consideration of the autonomy of patients whose circumstances make them particularly vulnerable. Even more deeply, the experiences of illness and announcement are at the ontological level, as shown above. It is all the more important to encourage the affected persons to express their will. Actually, it is up to the patients to decide if and when they want to have the information. These specific announcements are therefore intended to become a place of their *empowerment*.

9.2.3   The Role of Emotions

Physicians are meant to define the data to be communicated, to deliver information with respect for patient choices and tactfulness given the proven sensitivity to negative information. Obviously, these are risky communication situations, hence the need for ethical guidelines. As a result, the practitioners' empathic personal qualities, even when high-level, are not always sufficient, and the risk of burnout must be addressed if they do not also rely on learned communication techniques. Alongside tiredness, the specialisation of care with the technical evolution of medical practice and problems caused by economic costs, uncontrolled emotions can exhaust physicians and cause negligence or carelessness (Svandra 2009). In addition, empathy produces a wide range of attitudes from indifference to emotional invasion (Pacherie 2004). In fact, negative information impacts both the deliverer and the receiver. So, it is an issue for the therapeutic alliance, in itself complex, dynamic and multidimensional (Bordin 1979), that makes sense at the level of the relationship itself, regardless of the technical dimensions of the treatments (Bioy and Bachelart 2010). Yet, when the relationship between doctor and patient is correctly maintained, it is in itself therapeutic (Martin et al. 2000).

The point to consider here is the place given to emotions. Emotions may encourage us to act to solve a problem, but can be harmful if they make us act irrationally. On the one hand, we must be careful not to be ruled by them, but on the other hand, we have to be aware that they reveal our values, and they can alert us to our commitment to the main principles when they are at risk (Le Coz 2007). On the caregiver's side, autonomy is associated with respect, beneficence with compassion, non-maleficence with fear (Le Coz 2007). On the patient's side, lack of respect leads to indignation. In the context of the announcement, they certainly have a psycho-affective but above all an ethical dimension. Hence it is an important issue for the education of physicians not to denigrate emotions, to learn to identify their own feelings, and to deal with them in order to improve their relationships with patients (Marin and Worms 2015).

In an ethical approach that is concerned with the *caring* for patients, a genuine trusting relationship is based on a holistic view of the patient. The following questions: "What does the patient want?"; "How does the patient feel?"; "What does the doctor know about what the patient wants and how the patient feels?"; "How should one position oneself in relation to the patient and other physicians?", should precede the announcement. Moreover, the impact of false-positive test results and overdiagnosis on the patients' decision-making capacity and potentially on their physical and mental health must be taken into account. In communicating risks, benefits and uncertainties, personalised information is required, as is the case in breast cancer screening care (Ferretti et al. 2017).

Furthermore, it is also necessary that time and space be provided to promote a detailed understanding of the situation in all its aspects, in order to communicate in a manner that is suitable to the context. Only if this is achieved can the stress of negative information be overcome on both sides and a trusting relationship between the nuclear doctor and the patient established in an effective and appropriate way.

9.3 Implication for Practice and Training

9.3.1 Current Situations

Nuclear physicians and radiologists engage in challenging and stressful patient communication interactions. Before committing to such interactions, the nuclear physician/radiologist should be aware of:

1. The questions raised by the clinician and the potential therapeutic options according to the various results of the imaging study.
2. The performance of the imaging study in each specific situation. A prime example is the limited value of ^{18}F-FDG PET/CT in endocrine malignancies that do not rule out any active disease despite a negative finding.
3. The wish of the patient to get the result/report of the imaging test. In our opinion, except in very specific situations that would require the hospitalisation of the patient or the rapid booking of an appointment with a specialist, the breaking of bad news should be solely for patients who choose to have the results of their scan immediately afterwards.

The more comfortable situation for communicating imaging results is achieved when the imaging study is considered as highly reliable in a given situation and fails to identify any abnormality. Another situation that can be managed with limited stress is observed when the patient is perfectly aware of his disease and staging and the imaging study is concordant with the previous reports or expected results. All other situations can be very challenging and would require specific training.

In the US radiologists and imaging specialists do not give results to patients, but rather send them to the referring physician i.e. the oncologist. In France, patient information is ruled by regulatory and non-regulatory obligations. Cancer care plans emphasize the need to listen to patients and for quality information and support to be provided to them. However, these obligations remain non-specific and there is no consensus or guidelines on the modalities and content of communicating medical information to patients. In addition, each medical speciality has its own specific features. Furthermore, it has not been established that the imaging physician's participation in the announcement helps the patients cope with their illness.

Thus, the lack of specific recommendations about making an imaging announcement and the uncertainty about the real impact of such an approach partly explain the heterogeneity of practices. The papers of Tondeur et al. about the role played by nuclear medicine physicians in the transmission of radioisotope examination results to patients show that there are no official recommendations in 7 countries out of the 32 included in their study (Tondeur and Ham 2000a). Moreover, 70% of Belgian nuclear physicians adapt their attitude to the clinical situation of the patient (Tondeur and Ham 2000b). Finally, most of the Belgian nuclear doctors (90.5%) believe that an imaging doctor should never communicate a result to the patient, except in certain specific situations (Tondeur and Ham 2002).

Thus, the participation of nuclear medicine physicians in the announcement complies with regulatory requirements, but it must be implemented in a sustained institutional approach and carried out by the healthcare staff. In fact, rather than national guidelines it is more a question of the attitudes specific to each service, particularly dependent on the motivation of the caregivers. The most important thing is that the chosen attitude is approved by the whole team and a coherent care plan carried out. Frequent changes should be avoided. These changes could effectively destabilize patients who are repeatedly examined during their medical management. It also requires specific resources dedicated to this activity.

9.3.2 Teaching Strategies

There is a paucity of educational curricula on interpersonal and communication skills in imaging (Smith et al. 2012).

One of the proposed approaches would be to set up pre-announcement consultations in order to prepare patients to handle information pertaining to their health while consulting their referring physician, especially those patients asking for their results. For maximum empathy and efficacy, these consultations should take place in a dedicated space with trained and motivated personnel with an awareness of ethical and moral issues and any relevant cultural differences which might affect the practitioner-patient communication exchange. In order to meet these requirements, it is therefore important to organize specific training programs dedicated to the announcement of results. These programs would provide communication tools and strategies for delivering terrible news to patients.

However, research is still required to determine ideal methods of educating senior-level physicians and residents on the communication of test results. Role-play scenarios could represent a very suitable method for teaching such issues. Students would be placed in artificially created situations (Granry and Moll 2012). This pedagogical approach could certainly be based on repetition and standardisation, but to provide added ethical value it requires the implementation of authentic relational ethics supported by specific communication skills. Role-plays provide an opportunity for students to confront multidisciplinary practice contexts, to practice interprofessional collaboration, and to familiarise themselves with the main communicational pitfalls they may encounter in their daily practice (Tesnière and Fleury 2017).

To reinforce the integration of ethical principles into everyday practice, several scenarios that may arise in a nuclear medicine practice could be presented in the setting of role-plays with discussion of ethical dilemmas and suggested resolutions. The following represent some examples which could be effective.

A patient who suspects the recurrence of disease undergoes PET/CT imaging 5 years after initial management. The scan reveals evidence that the disease has recurred. They would like a report of the PET study.

A patient with a previous history of colon cancer has a large intensely hot lesion in the liver, consistent with metastasis. However, the liver MRI scan was interpreted as "classic for haemangioma" (a benign tumour). They would like to have the results of the PET/CT.

A patient had a metastatic disease on PET/CT imaging. However, a recent complete imaging work-up described only a localised disease susceptible to possible surgical treatment with curative intent. They would like a report of the PET study. They are not due to see their doctor for 4 more weeks.

9.3.3 Ethical Issues Around Role-Playing

In the training of students, their attention should be drawn to the context of the announcement itself, as well as the expectations that the patient can express verbally, namely speech and choice of words, but also to the expectations and emotions expressed in non-verbal communication, including the tone of voice, gestures, attitudes etc. From the point of view of communication ethics, the main difficulty lies in situations of mismatch between the announcement and what is expected or hoped for: unexpected announcement of cancer, relapse of an illness, severe decompensation that redirects the cure project towards palliative care. Students will also become aware that good news is very emotionally charged too and can lead to inappropriate behaviour. These situations include the announcement of remission, the diagnosis of cancer ruled out without finding any cause for the symptoms. When imaging and biology reveal nothing abnormal and physical suffering remains unexplained, professionals are confronted by the limitations of such examinations. By defensive reaction, they may reject or denigrate what the patient's says (Harrus-Révidi 2008). On this last point, it is important to stress the impact of the practitioner's recognition of the patient's psychological, emotional, and moral suffering, regardless of the physical cause of the disease, whether the cause is other than cancer or whether the disorders and symptoms are psychogenic. Authentic support for vulnerable people benefits from being experienced and understood in the exposure to other people, even when their autonomy seems afflicted (Pelluchon 2009).

In the care relationship, it is the recognition of humanity and the otherness of the person with whom we are dealing that are at stake. Role-playing is an opportunity to strengthen the participants' moral *ethos*, i.e. their attitude, their way of behaving, their inclination to relate to others in an adjusted, equitable, empathic way, and to reinforce their sense of responsibility. The aim is for students to gain flexibility in communication situations in order to better address the specificity of the ethical approach, because ethics help to navigate the route of least harm when faced with uncertainty. Students should also keep in mind the main principles of medical care: autonomy, dignity, integrity and vulnerability. At the time of the announcement, patients present themselves in all their vulnerability. The announcement can be understood as the moment of the encountering of the "face" of the Other, in the sense that the philosopher Levinas understands it (Levinas 1984, 1991). Indeed, the face of the Other is beyond representation, since "It's when you see a nose, eyes, a forehead, chin, and you can describe them, that you consider the others as objects. The best way to encounter the Other is not even to notice the colour of their eyes". According to Levinas: "The face is the reality par excellence, where someone does not show their qualities". The face-to-face encounter reveals the Other's absolute alterity. Because of their radical otherness, transcending the Self, the very humanity of the Other is evident in their ethical priority. Due to the infinity of the Other, the face imposes a high degree of responsibility for the Other on the Self, and specifically here on physicians.

The perception of disease and in particular cancer, retains negative connotations in our societies. Medical imaging is playing an increasingly important role in patient management, particularly in oncology. Regardless of their reliability, the impact of the results of these examinations on patients is considerable, and patients are keen on enquiring about the results on the day of the examination. This makes it a crucial moment, emotionally very charged, with consequences on the patients' adherence to their cure project. The communication of the results reveals ethical issues, related to the respect of the main principles shared by the medical community, such as autonomy, integrity, respect for the human person, and consideration of the persons' vulnerability. When delivering medical information from nuclear imaging "face-to-face", in philosophical and ethical dimensions, the physician can establish a trusting relationship with the patient, on the condition that the negative effects of uncontrolled emotions are overcome while being attentive to the positive aspects of these emotions. Ethical purpose in communication implies being attentive to the individuality of others, their expectations, capacities, and weaknesses – this being understood, it is up to the patient to choose what they want to know, according to the recognition of their rights and autonomy. The question of working in collaboration with the rest of the patient's medical team is also important. Although breaking bad news is an essential ability for medical professionals, there is a paucity of educational curricula on interpersonal and communication skills in imaging. Research is still required to determine ideal methods of educating senior-level physicians and residents on communicating diagnostic imaging results. Role-play scenarios could represent an appropriate method to achieve this goal. Ethical and communication skills could also be added to post-degree university curricula of nuclear physicians via taught courses and seminars with the integration of role-playing as a teaching method. All could be coordinated at national and European level. We acknowledge that such a program would raise several important economic questions, especially regarding human resources and limited financial recognition compared to the increase in the number of imaging examinations. However, this approach could start in certain pilot institutions with physicians, nurses and radiographers motivated to train themselves in this methodology and it could subsequently spread to a larger number of institutions.

References

Assoun, Paul-Laurent. 2009. L'Image Médicale À l'Épreuve De La Psychanalyse, Le Fantasme Iconographique. *Recherches en Psychanalyse* 2 (8): 182–189. https://doi.org/10.3917/rep.008.0182.

Beauchamp, Tom L., and James F. Childress. 1979. *Principles of biomedical ethics*. New York: Oxford University Press.

Béranger, Jérôme, and Pierre Le Coz. 2012. Réflexion Éthique Sur La Pluridisciplinarité Et La Confidentialité De l'Information En Imagerie Médicale Via Les Nouvelles Technologies De L'Information Et La Communication. *Cancer et Radiothérapie* 16 (3): 215–218. https://doi.org/10.1016/j.canrad.2011.10.012.

Bioy, Antoine, and Maximilien Bachelart. 2010. L'Alliance Thérapeutique: Historique, Recherches Et Perspectives Cliniques. *Perspectives Psy* 49 (4): 317–325. https://www.cairn.info/revue-perspectives-psy-2010-4-page-317.htm.

Bordin, Edward S. 1979. The generalizability of the psychoanalytic concept of the working alliance. *Psychotherapy: Theory, Research, and Practice* 16 (3): 252–260. https://doi.org/10.1037/h0085885.

Bougnoux, Daniel. 2009. *Introduction Aux Sciences De La Communication*. Paris: PUF.

Canguilhem, Georges. 1966. *Le Normal Et Le Pathologique*. Paris: PUF.

Centre d'études et de recherche sanitaire et médico-sociale de Poitiers. 1990. *La Personne Humaine Face Au Développement Des Sciences Biomédicales. 200 Ans Après La Déclaration Des Droits De l'Homme Et Du Citoyen De 1789*. Paris: Librairie de la cour de cassation.

Delehanty, Megan. 2010. Why images? *Medicine Studies* 2 (3): 161–173. https://doi.org/10.1007/s12376-010-0052-2.

Escarpit, Robert. 1991. *L'Information Et La Communication, Théorie Générale*. Paris: Hachette.

Estival, Cécile. 2010. Imagerie Médicale Et Rapport Au Corps Dans Un Centre De Cancérologie. *Découvrir* 1 (8): 108–110. https://doi.org/10.3917/corp.008/0105.

Ferretti, G., A. Linkeviciute, and G. Boniolo. 2017. Comprehending and communicating statistics in breast cancer screening. Ethical implications and potential solutions. In *Medical ethics, prediction and prognosis: Interdipliplinary perspectives*, ed. M. Gadebusch-Bondio, F. Spöring, and J.-S. Gordon, 30–41. New York: Routledge.

Gillies, R.J., P.E. Kinahan, and H. Hricak. 2015. Radiomics: Images are more than pictures, they are data. *Radiology* 278 (2): 563–577. https://doi.org/10.1148/radiol.2015151169.

Gonzalez, Sandra, Eric Guedj, Stefano Fanti, Elisabetta Lalumera, Pierre Le Coz, and David Taïeb. 2018a. Delivering PET imaging results to cancer patients: Steps for handling ethical issues. *European Journal of Nuclear Medicine and Molecular Imaging* 45 (12): 2240–2241. https://doi.org/10.1007/s00259-018-4124-y.

Gonzalez, S., P. Le Coz, Tondeur Abdullah, Griffon Loundou, Baumstarck Colavolpe, Mundler Banardel, and D. Taieb. 2018b. How do nuclear medicine physicians deal with ethical aspects of communicating results to patients after PET performed for oncological indications? A French National Survey. *Ethics, Medicine and Public Health* 4: 43–50. https://doi.org/10.1016/j.jemep.2017.12.007.

Granry, Jean-Claude, and Marie-Christine Moll. 2012. *Haute Autorité de la Santé, Rapport De Mission État de l'Art (National Et International) En Matière de Pratiques De Simulation Dans Le Domaine De La Santé, France*. https://www.has-sante.fr/portail/upload/docs/application/pdf/2012-01/simulation_en_sante_-_rapport.pdf.

Gusdorf, Georges. 1952. *La Parole*. Paris: PUF.

Harrus-Révidi, Gisèle. 2008. La Radiographie, Une Image Du Soi Inconnu. *L'Esprit du temps, Champs psychosomatique* 4 (52): 7–15. https://doi.org/10.3917/cpsy.052.0007.

Jankelevitch, Vladimir. 1966. *La Mort*. Paris: Flammarion.

Joyce, Kelly A. 2008. *Magnetic appeal: MRI and the myth of transparency*. Ithaca: Cornell University Press.

Kemp, Peter, and Jacob Rendtorff. 2000. Basic ethical principle in bioethics and biolaw: Report to the European Commission of the BIOMED Project basic ethical principles. In *Bioethics and biolaw 1995–1998*. Copenhagen/ Barcelona: Centre for Ethics and Law/Institut Borja de Bioètica.

Kemp, Peter, Rendtorff Jacob, and Niels Mattsson Johansen. 2000. *Four ethical principles*. Copenhagen: Rhodos International Science and Art Publisher, Centre for Ethics and Law.

Krupinski, Elizabeth A. 2010. Current perspectives in medical image perception. *Attention, Perception, & Psychophysics* 72 (5): 1205–1217. https://doi.org/10.3758/APP.72.5.1205.

Le Coz, Pierre. 2007. *Petit Traité De La Décision Médicale*. Paris: Seuil.

Levinas, Emmanuel. 1984. *Éthique Et Infini, Dialogues Avec Philippe Nemo*. Paris: Fayard.

———. 1991. *Totalité Et Infini*. Paris: Le Livre de Poche.

Marin, Claire. 2008a. *Hors De Moi*. Paris: Éditions Allia.

———. 2008b. *Violence De La Maladie, Violence De La Vie*. Paris: Colin.

———. 2014. *La Maladie, Catastrophe Intime*. Paris: PUF.

Marin, Claire, and Frédéric Worms. 2015. *À Quel Soin Se Fier ?: Conversations Autour De Winnicott*. Paris: PUF.

Martin, D.J., J.P. Garske, and M.K. Davis. 2000. Relation of the therapeutic alliance with outcome and other variables: A meta-analytic review. *Journal of Consulting and Clinical Psychology* 68 (3): 438–450. https://doi.org/10.1037/0022-006X.68.3.438.

Masson, Céline. 2007. L'Image En Médecine: Us Et Abus. L'Image N'Est Pas La Réalité. *Cliniques Méditerranéennes* 76 (2): 61–75. https://doi.org/10.3917/cm.076.0061.

Narayan, A., S. Dromi, A. Meeks, E. Gomez, and B. Lee. 2018. Breaking bad news: A survey of radiology residents' experiences communicating results to patients. *Current Problems in Diagnostic Radiology* 47 (2): 80–83. https://doi.org/10.1067/j.cpradiol.2017.04.011.

Pacherie, Elisabeth. 2004. L'Empathie Et Ses Degrés. In *L'Empathie*, ed. A. Berthoz and G. Jorland, 149–181. Paris: Odile Jacob.

Pelluchon, Corinne. 2009. *L'Autonomie Brisée: Bioéthique Et Philosophie*. Paris: PUF.

Potier, Rémy. 2007. L'Imagerie Médicale À l'Épreuve Du Regard. Enjeux éthiques D'Une Clinique Face À L'Image. *Cliniques méditerranéennes* 76 (2): 77–90. https://doi.org/10.3917/cm.076.0077.

———. 2012. L'Imagerie Médicale Dans La Relation De Soin Enjeux Psychiques Et Éthiques. *Revue Laennec* 60 (4): 40–46. https://doi.org/10.3917/lae.124.0040.

Ricœur, Paul. 1990. *Soi-Même Comme Un Autre*. Paris: Seuil.

———. 1995. *Le Juste I*. Paris: Éditions Esprit.

———. 2004. *Parcours De La Reconnaissance*. Paris: Stock.

———. 2007. *Vivant Jusqu'À La Mort*. Paris: Seuil.

Salaün, P.Y., R. Abgral, O. Malard, S. Querellou-Lefranc, G. Quere, M. Wartski, R. Coriat, E. Hindie, D. Taieb, A. Tabarin, A. Girard, J.F. Grellier, I. Brenot-Rossi, D. Groheux, C. Rousseau, D. Deandreis, J.L. Alberini, C. Bodet-Milin, E. Itti, O. Casasnovas, F. Kraeber-Bodere, P. Moreau, A. Philip, C. Balleyguier, A. Luciani, and F. Cachin. 2020. Good clinical practice recommendations for the use of PET/CT in oncology. *European Journal of Nuclear Medicine and Molecular Imaging* 47 (1): 28–50. https://doi.org/10.1007/s00259-019-04553-8.

Smith, K.V., J. Witt, J.A. Klaassen, C. Zimmerman, and A.-L. Cheng. 2012. High-fidelity simulation and legal/ethical concepts: A transformational learning experience. *Nursing Ethics* 19 (3): 390–398. https://doi.org/10.1177/0969733011423559.

Svandra, Philippe. 2009. *Le Soignant Et La Démarche Éthique*. Paris: Etsem.

Tassy, S., P. Le Coz, and B. Wickler. 2008. Current knowledge in moral cognition can improve medical ethics. *Journal of Medical Ethics* 34 (9): 679–682. https://doi.org/10.1136/jme.2006.018812.

Terrou, Fernand. 1962. *L'Information*. Paris: PUF.

Tesnière, Antoine, and Cynthia Fleury. 2017. La Simulation En Santé Pour Mieux Soigner. *Soins* 62 (820): 56–59.

The Nuremberg Code. 1947. In *Doctors of infamy: The story of Nazi medical crimes*, ed. A. Mitscherlich and F. Mielke, xxiii–xxv. New York: Schuman, 1949.

Tondeur, Marianne, and Hyeseung Ham. 2000a. Should nuclear medicine physicians give the results of radioisotope examinations directly to patients? *Nuclear Medicine Communications* 21 (8): 781–783. https://doi.org/10.1097/00006231-200008000-00013.

———. 2000b. Should we give the examination results to the patients? *Revue Médicale de Bruxelles* 21 (2): 95–98.

———. 2002. Transmission of examination results to patients: Opinion of referring physicians and patients. *Acta Clinica Belgica* 57 (3): 129–133. https://doi.org/10.1179/acb.2002.028.

United Nations. 1948. *Universal Declaration of Human Rights*. https://www.un.org/en/universal-declaration-human-rights/index.html.

Van Dijk, José. 2005. *The transparent body: A cultural analysis of medical imaging*. Seattle: University of Washington Press.

Walker, Tom. 2009. What principlism misses. *Journal of Medical Ethics* 35: 229–231. https://doi.org/10.1136/jme.2008.027227.

Weindling, Paul. 2001. The origins of informed consent: The international scientific commission on medical war crimes, and The Nuremberg Code. *Bulletin of History of Medicine* 75 (1): 37–71.

World Medical Association. 2013. Declaration of Helsinki: Ethical principles for medical research involving human subjects. *Journal of the American Medical Association* 310 (20): 2191–2194. https://doi.org/10.1001/jama.2013.281053.

Wunenburger, Jean-Jacques. 1997. *Philosophie De L'Image*. Paris: PUF.

Printed in the United States
by Baker & Taylor Publisher Services